Your Heart and How to Live with It

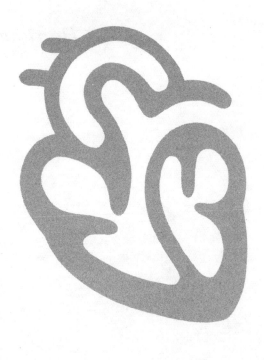

Your Heart and

How to Live with It

LAWRENCE E. LAMB, M.D.

New York / THE VIKING PRESS

Library of Congress catalog card number: 69-15662
Printed in U.S.A.

Second printing November 1969

Grateful acknowledgment is made to the American
Heart Association, Inc. for their permission to
use the diet plan from *The Way to a Man's Heart*
Copyright © American Heart Association, 1968, and
for the use of the illustrations on pages 229 and 230.

Foreword

ALMOST EVERYONE in the United States and in most of the industrialized countries of the world today either has disease of the heart or blood vessels or has a member of the immediate family or close friend with such a disorder. Heart and vascular diseases are the foremost medical problems of our time.

There are things which each person can do to prevent the complications of heart and vascular diseases. There is much that can be done to improve one's health even after a heart attack. This book was written with the hope that the reader will gain enough knowledge to be able to avoid death or disability from these disorders.

Sooner or later most individuals are confronted with the problem of a person who has lost consciousness either from a simple faint or because of a heart attack. The person may need artificial circulation which you can provide if you know how. Heart transplants, artificial hearts, modern coronary-care units, and computers will not help the person who drops dead. Unless prompt assistance is available—usually from a nonmedical person—life is over. The sensational events surrounding the efforts to develop an artificial heart or the drama of a few heart transplants are insignificant compared to the big picture of heart disease. A great problem in the industrial nations of the world is the millions of people dying annually from heart disease and millions of others who are crippled or disabled each year by this greatest medical problem of all time.

Everyone needs to know what the important features of diet are as protection against heart and vascular disease—the importance of cigarettes, coffee, and alcohol. The entire population is almost totally ignorant concerning the effects of sexual activity on the heart and its relationship to heart disease—or how to maintain adequate heart function to preserve sexual capacity.

Exercise is said to be good for the heart—but why? It can kill as well as help, and exercise quacks are taking a toll nearly equal to the toll of diet quacks. You need to know the proper use of exercise to gain its benefits without becoming its victim.

Recent confidence that something can be done to prevent heart disease has been underscored by the National Board of Health and Welfare of Sweden and the National Medical Board of Finland, making official recommendations on May 3, 1968, to the public concerning diet and exercise. In the United States, the American Heart Association has recommended changes in national dietary habits.

I firmly believe that if the public at large understood the magnitude of the problem, and followed the principles outlined in this book, the national problem of heart and vascular disease could be significantly reduced—perhaps to minor importance. By educating one's self, and then being a leader by example, all readers can help themselves and their loved ones. For this reason this may be the most important book you ever read in your lifetime.

1969   LAWRENCE E. LAMB, M.D.

Contents

Your Heart and How to Live with It

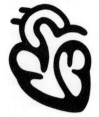

CHAPTER I

What You Don't Know Can Kill You

HAVE YOU EVER wondered how you will die? If you are an American, there is a greater than fifty-per-cent chance that you will die of a circulatory disease—a disease of the heart or blood vessels. If you are an adult male, or a female approaching the menopause, you probably already have disease of the arteries to your heart or other vital organs. Disease of the heart and blood vessels kills more Americans every year than all other diseases and accidents combined. The great killer is not unsafe automobiles, highway accidents, or other forms of violence. It is not tuberculosis or other infectious diseases. The great killer is heart disease. In the entire history of mankind no plague, pestilence, disaster, or epidemic has ever seriously rivaled this champion of all time. In the United States, in 1963, over one million people died of cardiovascular diseases. The American Heart Association estimates that 1,059,400 of the 1,946,100 deaths in the United States occurring in 1969 can be attributed to cardiovascular disease. This is fifty-four per cent of all deaths.

The brilliant advances in medicine have helped a few, while the specter of death, disability, and tragedy for Mr. and Mrs. Average America remains unsolved and unchecked. Each year, more and more knowledge is gained in reducing the probabilities of being disabled or killed from circulatory diseases. Much of this knowledge has not been applied. Many facets of everyday living habits do have a direct bearing upon the likelihood of having heart disease. There is a great deal that the individual person can do for himself in delaying or preventing death or disability from heart disease—if he knows how. This includes weight control, adequate exercise, and general hygienic living.

Failure to control the great killer does not minimize the many advances that have been made by medicine in the past several decades, particularly in the prevention of rheumatic heart disease and improved surgical techniques. Heart attacks, however, are appreciably more frequent today than they were ten years ago. Medical problems of the American and European nations have changed; the major health problems of fifty years ago were tuberculosis and the other infectious diseases. Pneumonia and other severe infections had to be treated without the aid of antibiotics or other modern drugs that are now commonplace. Weight loss seldom was the result of dietary control, but more often suggested underlying tuberculosis. When unexplained weight loss occurred, people feared that tuberculosis had condemned another to a life of invalidism and eventual death.

The Mystery of Unexplained Chest Pain

Although it was not known that heart disease could cause chest and arm pain, early accounts of unexplained illness were typical of disorders that have more recently been attributed to the heart. Physicians were puzzled by occasional illnesses such as that of the Earl of Clarendon, Lord High Chancellor of England. The Earl was seized by sharp pain in the left arm, lasting "half a quarter of an hour" of such severity that he turned pale. In 1670 the Earl commented that he had passed the pangs of death, and he should die in one of those fits. The account states that he had the "image of death" constantly before him. Four years later, at the age of sixty-five, after hurrying to meet his brother, he was again seized by a pain in his arm and dropped dead.

In the latter part of the eighteenth century the famous British physician William Heberden, referred to by his colleagues as "the last of our learned physicians," recorded his observations of "Pectoris Dolor" (chest pain). It was he who coined the term *angina pectoris* for this disorder. He noted its onset with physical exertion and its eventual progression until it also occurred at rest. He observed that the disorder had not had a name or place in medical writings and that he could offer no treatment for this strange malady. Although he described the symptoms clearly, he did not demonstrate that they were caused by heart disease. In the light of current interest in the relationship between exercise and heart disease it is interesting that, according to Dr. Heberden, one patient "set himself a task of sawing wood for half an hour every day, and was nearly cured."

In 1910 physicians were beginning to ascribe recurrent episodes of intermittent chest pain, known as angina pectoris, to heart disease. The famous physician Sir William Osler described the prototype of today's victim. He noted that it was "not the delicate, neurotic person" who had this disorder but "the robust, the vigorous in mind and body, the keen and ambitious man, the indicator of whose engines is always at 'full speed ahead.'" Osler thought there was a type of individual who experienced these disorders and described him as a "well 'set' man of from forty-five to fifty years of age, with military bearing, iron grey hair, and florid complexion."

Chest pain and other manifestations of a heart attack (*myocardial infarction*) were not identified with obstruction of a coronary artery until the early 1900s. Two German physicians, W. P. Obrastzow and N. D. Stroschesko, made the important correlation between the patient's illness and the changes in the heart.

The first accurate description of the events of a heart attack by an American physician is attributed to Dr. James B. Herrick, who made his observations as recently as 1912. The illness he described of a fifty-five-year-old man, with no previous evidence of disease, is now a commonplace episode in American life. One hour after a moderately full meal the man had severe pain in the lower portion of the central chest. Shortly after this he was nauseated, and thought he had eaten something which disagreed with him. The pain was severe and lasted more than three hours. The man became pale and sweaty, his pulse was feeble and his heart rate rapid. There were other signs which were described. In less than three days after the onset of his illness, he was dead. An examination of the heart demonstrated a clot in one of the major arteries to the heart muscle. Although considered a medical rarity in 1912, this is now a common end to the American executive's career. In little more than fifty years the rare has become first commonplace and finally the expected.

The Greatest Threat to Your Life

Since those early observations of diseases of the arteries to the heart, many major improvements have come about in the control and prevention of heart disease. The scourge of syphilis which may affect the heart and its valves, was once a frequent cause of heart disease. Since the advent of penicillin, however, early detection and treatment of syphilis in the United States has nearly eradicated cardiac complications from venereal disease. Rheumatic fever— once a commonplace cause for destruction of the valves of the heart, even in the very young—has become a minor disease of infrequent occurrence. While this disease still exists, large specialized hospitals for children with rheumatic fever are no longer needed in the United States. Many hospitals that previously were designed for this purpose are now filled by children with other disorders. Many children born with cardiac defects have had complete or partial surgical corrections of these abnormalities. Despite these achievements the great killer has gone unchecked; and if you are an American, heart disease is the greatest threat to your life, health, and future happiness.

Not only does one out of two Americans die of circulatory disease but many individuals are significantly disabled during the course of their lives by heart disease. Each year there are over twelve million Americans who develop complications of circulatory diseases other than death. These include such problems as intermittent chest pain, nonfatal heart attacks, heart failure, and many other disorders. Of this large number of people, approximately two million are severely or permanently disabled.

In 1963 it was estimated that one out of every four Americans between the ages of eighteen and eighty had a medical problem (symptoms or findings on medical examination) that was thought to be caused by heart disease. It is heart and vascular disease that has prevented people from dying of old age in this century of medical miracles.

A disease of such magnitude is not without its economic impact. There are, of course, the expenditures related to hospitalization, nursing care, physicians, medicines, and the gamut of modern-day medical care. Aside from this, there is the loss of the wage earner's capacity—not only during critical illnesses but often for months or years later. There is also the permanent loss of wage earnings to the families of those who die. An estimate of the economic cost of vascular disease in the United States in 1963 was approximately twenty-five billion dollars, or an expenditure equal to the annual budget of the Vietnam war. These staggering economic costs are only part of the picture. It is cardiovascular disease that frequently removes the father or young husband from the family circle, or cuts short his promising career.

Circulatory diseases are the real reason that life expectancy for men in the United States has not increased over the last twenty years. In this regard, the United States is far behind many other nations of the world. The simple truth is that in the United States, the life expectancy for the American male has not changed during the past twenty years despite an increase in federal expenditures for biomedical research from one million to one billion dollars. There is a strong suspicion that although medical research has brought about many marvelous and extraordinary advances, the factors that are important in preventing the devastating effects of heart disease are in contrast commonplace and mundane.

Are You Too Young to Have a Heart Attack?

Despite the fact that the great killer—vascular disease—was first described in middle-aged men, it soon became common to consider a heart attack or a stroke, not as a disease, but rather as a manifestation of the aging process. It was recognized that rheumatic heart disease often struck the young, and syphilitic heart disease was known to be the culprit in certain cases as were other infections associated with heart disease, but the heart attack and the stroke were often ascribed to simple aging. Prior to World War II there were sporadic reports of young men under forty years of age who had genuine heart attacks of the type now recognized as commonplace. Some of these were probably caused by syphilis of the heart and inflammation of the coronary arteries. Occasional cases were even noted under twenty years of age. The ubiquitous nature of heart disease was becoming manifest.

During World War II an opportunity existed to observe the incidence of heart attacks in relatively young men in the armed services. From material collected by the Army Institute of Pathology, Dr. Wallace Yater and others amassed 866 cases of young men between the ages of eighteen and thirty-nine who had heart attacks.

Of these, 450 had been in apparent good health up until the time of their death. Characteristically, death occurred suddenly with little or no warning. Examination of the heart demonstrated typical changes in the major arteries to the heart muscle. In this large series, sixty-four of the men were between the ages of eighteen and twenty-four. Over two hundred of the men were twenty-nine years of age or less. Even though it was apparent that the heart attack was less common in young men below the age of thirty-five, these studies did much to demonstrate that the heart attack was in fact a disease, not simply a manifestation of aging.

Autopsies and other studies through the period of World War II confirmed that coronary atherosclerosis (fatty deposits in the coronary arteries) began in some individuals at a very early age. How often it occurred still remained a matter of speculation.

The Korean War created an opportunity to determine how many apparently healthy young men had coronary atherosclerosis. Autopsies were performed on a number of the young soldiers killed in combat at an average age of twenty-two. When the major arteries to the heart were opened, evidence of disease was apparent. The accumulation of fatty deposits in the arterial wall that ultimately leads to its occlusion was present in over seventy-seven per cent of these young men. In ten per cent the process had already occluded over seventy per cent of the opening of one or more of the major arteries. These diseased arteries were not those of sedentary middle-aged men, but those of young, active, apparently healthy individuals, representing a group of Americans presumably in better than average health. Despite all external evidence of good health, heart disease had already begun its deadly process.

In other studies of individuals in successively older groups, the disease increased in frequency and severity with increasing age. For this reason it is almost certain that if the coronary arteries of most American men past the age of thirty were examined, one would find visible evidence that the occlusive process had begun to strangle the blood supply to the heart muscle. The silent sickness continues undetected by usual medical examination (although it can sometimes be detected by examinations of the coronary arteries)—since in its early stages it does not compromise the work of the heart. Usually heart disease progresses until it damages the heart, produces sudden severe chest pain, or causes sudden death, before its presence is detected.

There is a growing body of evidence that disease of the coronary arteries is increasing in young men. Autopsy studies have demonstrated that in all age groups of the adult male, fatty deposits are more frequent and severe now than twenty-five years ago. Men thirty years of age have more disease than forty-year-old men used to have. The forty-year-old men have as much or more disease than fifty-year-old men had a generation ago.

In January 1968, it was reported to the medical profession that the leading cause for unexpected sudden death in young men was coronary artery disease. In 275 consecutive autopsies in New York City, in men twenty to forty-five years of age, coronary artery disease was the cause of death in thirty-eight per cent of the group.

In recent years, annual examinations of United States Air Force flying personnel demonstrated that a surprising number of silent heart attacks had occurred between successive evaluations. These individuals had survived unrecognized heart attacks while continuing their usual military duties, which in certain instances included flying high-performance jet aircraft. Some of the young men who had heart attacks were in their early twenties.

Age and Heart Attacks

Despite the evidence of coronary artery disease in young men, heart attacks are relatively uncommon before the age of thirty. The frequency of complications of coronary artery disease, such as heart attacks, increases progressively with age. Heart attacks are not rare in young men between thirty and thirty-five years of age, but beyond age thirty-five the likelihood of heart attacks increases sharply. The American men most susceptible to heart attacks are those between fifty and sixty years of age, and after age sixty there is a sharp decrease in the percentage of individuals having heart attacks. In recent studies of Army personnel it was determined that, among diseases, the leading cause of death was coronary artery disease, at an average age of forty-three years.

Although the atherosclerotic disease process begins early in life, it is not until it suddenly occludes the blood flow to an area of the heart muscle that a heart attack (infarction) occurs. Such an occlusion can occur at any time in a diseased artery. The most effective prevention of the heart attack probably begins early in life as opposed to efforts made after the disease has achieved extensive proportions. A great deal can be done to improve the heart and prevent progression of disease even after surviving a heart attack.

Some Women Get a Break

Women are not immune to heart disease, but there is a distinct difference in their susceptibility to heart attacks. In white American females, prior to the menopause, there usually is no significant evidence of coronary artery disease unless the woman has high blood pressure, kidney disease, or diabetes. The occurrence of heart attacks appears to be increasing in American women. Between the ages of thirty and forty-five years men have heart attacks about thirteen times as often as women. From forty-five to sixty-two years of age the ratio of heart attacks between men and women is two to one. After age sixty-five, the frequency of heart attacks between Caucasian men and women is about the same.

The sex difference in the rate of heart attacks among Caucasian men and women is not observed in American Negroes. Coronary artery disease is almost as common in the American Negro female as in the American Negro male and more than twice as frequent as in the Caucasian American female. There are other differences too. Whereas the Caucasian female often has recurrent chest pain without a full-blown heart attack, the Negro female is apt to have the more severe form of heart attack usually seen in the male.

The difference in frequency of heart attacks between white males and females has not been adequately explained. It is thought that the female hormones offer a degree of protection against some of the multiple factors which lead to disease of the coronary arteries. The differences in smoking habits, exposure to the stress of competitive drive in modern society, and perhaps anatomical differences in the coronary arteries themselves, all have been cited as reasons for the sexual difference. After a woman has gone through the menopause and ceases to create the same amount of female hormones, there is an acceleration of coronary artery disease. Women who have had artificial removal of their ovaries likewise demonstrate an increased frequency of coronary artery disease as compared to normal females in the same age group. Why American Negro women are so much more susceptible to coronary artery disease than Caucasian women remains an enigma. There are many factors other than sex that influence coronary artery disease. High blood pressure and kidney disease seem to be more common in young Negro women than in other American women and may be important factors.

Heart Disease Around the World

The fatty deposits in the walls of the arteries that cause most heart disease in the United States and Europe are almost unknown in many parts of the world. This observation strongly suggests that the early appearance of such deposits is directly related to the differences in living habits between the developed and underdeveloped nations, so-called "have" and "have-not" nations, terms that apply equally as well to the presence or absence of fatty disease of the arteries among their populations.

The Bantu of Uganda have been frequently studied medically. In one study of 6,500 Bantu autopsy specimens not a single example of the fatty deposits was found in the coronary arteries. Another study of one hundred Bantu and one hundred Americans of the same age and sex demonstrated that although half of the Americans had fatty deposits in the arteries of the heart, occluded arteries, and scars of the heart muscle from old heart attacks, the Bantu showed very little evidence of atherosclerosis. The only Bantu showing fatty deposits in the coronary arteries were men in the seventy-year-old group, and even then the changes were minimal.

Numerous studies of this type have been accomplished by different investigators, and in each instance the findings were the same—extensive disease in Americans and Europeans and minimal or no disease in the Bantu or other Africans of similar living patterns. The Bantu are vigorous people. Some of their best war dancers are strong men in their sixties and seventies. They have good teeth and bones—usually better than their European and American counterparts.

Similar observations were made in the rice-eating nations. For many years fatty degeneration of the arteries was considered almost nonexistent in China. Later autopsy studies demonstrated fatty deposits in the arteries of elderly Chinese, usually milder and occurring twenty years later than in the industrialized nations. The lean, sparsely eating peoples of India are also relatively free of diseased arteries, as are other Asians living the less abundant life.

In an interesting autopsy study of 150 Japanese civilians in Okinawa, only seven were found to have fatty deposits in the coronary arteries and those deposits were minimal. The islanders had been vigorous, well-developed people, but they were not fat and they had habitually eaten a low-fat diet of rice, vegetables, sweet potatoes, and soybeans with little or no meat.

It is tempting to attribute these geographic differences in heart disease to variations in susceptibility, but other studies indicate this is not the case. In Johannesburg, white prisoners who were jailed for long terms with the Bantu were fed the Bantu diet. Their symptoms and clinical evidence of coronary artery disease disappeared. An age-matched autopsy study of individuals of the same racial background in New Orleans and Costa Rica demonstrates the frequent presence of a significantly greater degree of coronary occlusion in the well-fed people of New Orleans than observed in the poor Costa Ricans.

Although many factors influence susceptibility to atherosclerosis, most geographic studies strongly implicate the diet as a leading factor. The lack of exercise, the sounds, smells, and frustrations of modern civilization may well contribute to the problem, but diet alone has been cited as the important factor in the living habits of the Rendille, a nomadic tribe of camel herders in northern Kenya. Far removed from the trappings of civilization, the everyday life of these nomadic people demands vigorous physical activity, yet they are afflicted by coronary artery disease and its complications almost as often as the urbanized European or American. Why is this so? Perhaps the answer is in what they eat. Their diet, like that of their civilized counterparts, contains thirty-five to forty per cent fat. This strongly suggests that correcting all the supposed ills of modern civilization will not thwart the great killer unless the diet is optimal.

The Jewish people are thought to be particularly prone to heart disease; however the primitive Yemenite Jews were found to be relatively free of disease until they were absorbed by the Israeli modern culture. Then they too developed fatty deposits in the arteries and were prone to heart attacks.

When individuals from less affluent cultures have been transplanted to western civilization and developed new living patterns, they exhibit a relatively high incidence of coronary artery disease. There are some exceptions to this general rule: Dr. Irvine Page reported that American Navaho Indians, living in Cleveland, Ohio—

despite twentieth-century American influences, diet, and habits—have a relatively low incidence of complications from coronary artery disease.

Caution must be exercised in evaluating the differences in the frequency of heart attacks in different regions of the world. It was once claimed that the Alaskan Eskimos had a low incidence of coronary artery disease. A careful review of these studies, however, indicated they involved Eskimo populations with very few individuals older than thirty years of age. The scope of the medical examinations was not sufficient to have identified fatty deposits in the coronary arteries. This type of pitfall in interpreting statistics leads to erroneous conclusions about variations in heart disease in different civilizations. It should be readily apparent that in those areas of the world in which life expectancy is thirty years or less, the frequency of heart attacks will necessarily be low. These comments are not applicable to the well-done anatomical studies that form the basis for most of the conclusions about the presence or absence of disease in different countries and in different cultures.

World War II provided some bonus information regarding factors related to atherosclerosis. During the German occupation of the Scandinavian countries and the Lowlands, the diet of the people was markedly restricted in calories and fat. The toll of heart disease dropped dramatically. In the postwar years, when old living habits were resumed, even more people had heart attacks than before the war years. German prisoners of war, held in Russia, were fed low-fat diets of less than eight per cent fat. Autopsy studies on hundreds of German prisoners showed clean, healthy coronary arteries, relatively free of fatty deposits. When the surviving prisoners returned to Germany after the war and resumed their previous diets, the frequency of heart disease soared.

Throughout most of the world the picture has been fairly consistent. Wherever life is easy and abundant the great killer finds man an easy prey. If life is hard and rich foods less abundant, man is spared from strokes, heart attacks, and other complications of fatty degeneration of the arteries.

The ravages of atherosclerosis are most often seen in the industrialized nations of western civilization. *The leading cause of death is heart disease in Australia, Canada, Denmark, Finland, France, Netherlands, Norway, Sweden, Switzerland, United Kingdom, United States, and West Germany.*

Heart disease other than atherosclerosis is common throughout the world. Rheumatic heart disease is perhaps more prevalent in the Philippines, Korea, and much of Asia today, than it is in the United States. In those nations in which modern medical management for the prevention of infectious diseases is not available, or where nutrition is deficient, other forms of heart disease are more common. In some of the poor people of Africa that subsist on very substandard diets, there are abnormal changes in the heart muscle. The lining of the inner surface of the heart becomes thickened and inelastic. These changes lead to abnormal function of the heart and eventually to heart failure.

Do You Like the Odds?

Despite the grim outlook associated with heart disease in the United States and other industrialized nations of the world, there are a number of practical things which can be done to thwart atherosclerosis. The real goal is to prevent heart attacks, prevent heart disease, and prevent strokes. The idea of developing an artificial heart is an exciting one, and transplanting a human heart, even with temporary success, is a glamorous achievement, but a more satisfactory goal is being able to maintain your own heart in a good functional capacity, thereby avoiding becoming part of these dramatic human experiments.

Much has been done in recent years to improve the outlook of the heart-attack patient who survives long enough to be admitted to the hospital. In some good hospitals, the death rate has dropped from approximately forty to twenty per cent. These still are not very good odds, and despite recent advancements it is obviously preferable not to need these services in the first place.

You Can Do It Yourself and You May Have To

At present there seems to be no definitive proof that disease of the coronary arteries can be completely prevented. There is, however, a great deal that can be done to avoid the complications of coronary artery disease, such as heart attacks. Some of these programs are of great use to the individual who has already sustained a heart attack and survived. In other instances these programs improve the likelihood that an individual can survive a heart attack.

In the main, these measures are related to the proper use of physical activity, proper diet, and proper living habits. These are all things which fall in the realm of every individual's control. They are facets of our lives which cannot be legislated. They are factors which cannot be changed by improving the size or capability of our hospitals and clinics.

It is important to remember that your doctor cannot tell you that you don't have heart disease even after examining you thoroughly. Atherosclerosis often is a silent killer. The gradual accumulation of fat deposits in the coronary arteries causes no changes in heart function that he can detect by physical examination, blood tests, usual x-ray studies, or electrocardiograms. Often the first real evidence of heart disease is a heart attack, and when this causes sudden death the first warning is also the last. The plain truth is that your doctor, regardless of how capable he is, usually cannot detect the presence of the silent killer until it is too late. To date he has not been very successful in preventing his patients from having a heart attack. Under these circumstances you may have to take steps yourself to prevent having an attack. Basically you can do more for yourself than your doctor can, if you know what to do. Only you can change your habits. Your doctor can't do it for you.

If you don't know the proper use of exercise and physical activity, the proper approach to diet and nutrition, as well as the important role that living patterns and habits play in causing heart disease—what you don't know can kill you.

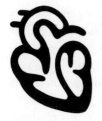

CHAPTER II

The Magnificent
Pump

THE HEART and blood vessels provide the body with a complex transport mechanism. The four-chambered heart is a pump, while the arteries and veins act as a plumbing system for the flow of blood. The circulating blood transports vital substances, such as oxygen, nutrients, and hormones to the cells. The blood stream carries the waste products of metabolism to the lungs, kidneys, and other organs that modify them or eliminate them from the body.

Fish and Fetus

The embryonic development of man's circulation is a remarkable feat of nature, each step mimicking the circulation of other living creatures. In the first three weeks of life, the small aggregate of human cells are bathed in the tissue fluids of the mother. As in primitive organisms, vital substances simply diffuse into the cells and waste products diffuse outward. The mother's circulation takes care of the rest. As the tiny embryo grows, it becomes more complex and requires its own individual transport system. By three weeks, an aggregate of specialized cells clump together near the head and a tubelike structure develops along the length of the embryo. The tube begins to grow and twist upon itself. The twisted tube develops first ridges and finally partitions that divide the newly formed heart into four main chambers.

While the heart is being formed, blood vessels begin to appear as individual segments throughout the developing embryo. The major blood vessels extending directly from the heart have loops between them called arches. These arches form a network of blood vessels similar to those seen in the fish to provide circulation to the gills—one of the developmental steps in the embryo linked to the theory of evolution. As the "fish stage" passes, the extra vessel loops degenerate or are used to form new routes for the developing vascular tree.

By six weeks, the human fetus has its own transportation system. While the fetus is sealed in the fluid-filled sac in the uterus, the lungs remain collapsed and all circulatory exchange of nutrients, gases, and waste products must be by way of the mother's blood stream. The baby's blood and the mother's blood exchange products across thin membranes in the placenta. The placental blood is shunted through the umbilical cord directly through the baby's liver to the fetal heart. Through structures that later close at birth, most of the blood is shunted through the baby's heart, directly into the circulation of the body, bypassing the collapsed fetal lungs.

The Right Heart

The heart is a four-chambered organ that serves as a reservoir and a pump for the circulating blood. After blood bathes the muscles, organs, and other tissues, it returns to the heart via two great veins, the superior vena cava from the upper body and the inferior vena cava from the lower body. Because the blood loses its oxygen and absorbs carbon dioxide the bright red color of fully oxygenated blood changes to a darker hue, imparting a bluish color to tissue as noted in the veins of the hand and elsewhere. The blood collects in the right atrial chamber of the heart.

The *right atrium* is a thin-walled, saclike structure situated at the top of the heart. The thin walls of the right atrium are lined with heart muscle, giving it the ability to contract and expel its contents at the proper moment.

Near the top of the right atrium, where the great veins enter the heart, there is a very tiny comma-shaped structure called the *sino-atrial node,* which is responsible for the heart rate. This specialized tissue is a cross between heart muscle and nerve tissue. It is the

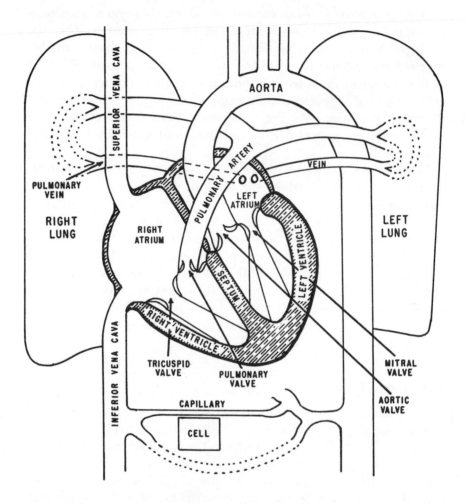

spark plug or pacemaker for the heart. Each time the pacemaker discharges, it changes its electrical state, stimulating electrical activity in the atrial muscle fibers causing the right atrium to contract. If the pacemaker fires frequently, the heart rate is rapid. If the rate of the pacemaker slows, the heart rate slows. The pacemaker is controlled by nerves from the spinal cord and brain. Nerve fibers directly from the brain tend to slow the heart, while those from the spinal cord tend to speed the heart. Their actions are integrated within the brain. When a person is excited, nerve impulses to the pacemaker increase the heart rate. In other instances, such as during breath holding, signals directly from the brain slow the heart rate. If the nerve fibers to the heart are cut, the pacemaker exhibits its own inherent rate, and through mechanisms that are not completely understood, responds to differences in pressure and volume within the heart itself.

At the bottom of the right atrial reservoir is a large opening into a second chamber called the *right ventricle.* The right ventricle is part of the thick muscular portion of the heart responsible for its main pumping action. At the opening between the right atrial reservoir and the right ventricle is the *tricuspid valve,* so called because it is composed of three leaflets or cusps. The valve is anchored at the outer circumference of the bottom of the right atrium. The free inner margins of the cusps are anchored by small cords, or stringlike structures, to muscular areas within the right ventricle. When the valve leaflets close, these three leaflets are stretched against the restraining cords like a sail in the wind. The three billowed sails close in apposition to each other, occluding the opening between the right atrial and ventricular cavities.

Blood accumulating in the right atrium gradually distends its walls. The right ventricular chamber begins to relax, permitting the tricuspid valve between the atrium and ventricle to open, so that blood flows freely from the atrial reservoir into the right ventricular chamber. Finally, the atrium contracts, squeezing the last of its blood into the right ventricular cavity.

The right ventricle lies immediately beneath the *sternum* (breastbone) in the lower central region of the chest. It is chiefly responsible for pumping blood to the lungs. As with the other chambers of the heart, when the muscular cavity is relaxed, or dilated, and filled with blood, it is said to be in *diastole*—in a state of dilation.

Near the tricuspid valve in the right atrium there is another specialized pacemaker called the *atrio-ventricular node* (A-V node). From this specialized structure a long pencil-like bundle of specialized tissue (the right bundle branch) extends into the right ventricle and terminates as fine filaments which infiltrate and ultimately stimulate the ventricular muscle mass. Another major network of connected fibers extends into the left side of the heart (the left bundle branch). This network electrically connects the atria to the ventricles. In many ways these structures are specialized nervous tissue—an electrical network used to stimulate different parts of the heart muscle.

The pumping action of the heart is so integrated that just after the right atrium has contracted, filling the right ventricle to its greatest extent, a stimulus passes from the ventricular pacemaker to cause contraction of the right ventricle. As the pressure increases in the right ventricle, the three flaps of the tricuspid valve close abruptly. The large pulmonary artery originating at the top or shoulder region of the right ventricular cavity carries all the blood to the lungs. At its opening is another valve, called the *pulmonary valve,* composed of three simple leaflets. While the ventricles are filling, this closed valve prevents blood from flowing backward from the lungs into the ventricle. As the pressure increases within the right ventricular chamber these valves open and blood is forced outward through them into the large pulmonary artery. Contraction continues until, under resting circumstances, about half of the blood in the right ventricle is ejected outward through the pulmonary artery into the lungs. Once the peak of the contraction of the ventricles has passed, the muscular wall begins to relax, causing the pressure in the right ventricular cavity to fall. The three cusps of the pulmonary valve snap shut, and once again the right ventricle begins to fill in preparation for its next contraction.

The large pulmonary artery divides into two main branches: one for the right lung and one for the left lung. The arteries then branch and diversify much like the trunk of a tree with its numerous branches and twigs. Through this system blood is carried to each of the individual air sacs of the lungs for the exchange of oxygen and carbon dioxide. The blood pumped by the right heart circulation is relatively low in oxygen content.

The Left Heart

After the gaseous exchanges have taken place between the blood and the lungs, all the blood is returned to the heart. The small vessels throughout the lung field gradually join to form four major veins. These all enter within a small area on the back wall of another saclike reservoir, called the *left atrium.* This structure is very much like the right atrium except that it is to the left and behind the right atrial structure. These two reservoirs constitute the top part of the heart and are divided from each other by a partition or septum. At the bottom of the left atrium is a large opening into the left ventricular cavity. The valve to this opening has only two leaflets or cusps and is called the *mitral valve*. This valve is of particular importance because it is frequently deformed by rheumatic fever. As a result of this process the valve may be scarred and obstructed, impeding flow of the blood through it. In other instances the valve may be partially destroyed, allowing blood to regurgitate freely into the left atrium when the valve should normally be closed. This valve was one of the earliest ones successfully repaired by surgery.

The mitral valve opens directly into a fourth chamber of the heart—the *left ventricle*. In the normal adult this is the heaviest and thickest portion of the heart. The left ventricle is directly connected to the right ventricle. The two ventricular cavities are separated by a partition called the ventricular septum. It is the left ventricular muscle mass that must do the greatest amount of work for the heart as the contraction of this muscle pumps blood through all of the body except the lungs. It must force the blood out under sufficient pressure to cause the flow of blood to the most distant regions of the body. In every sense it should be considered a working muscle.

Under normal circumstances the left atrial reservoir is filling with blood from the lungs while the right atrial reservoir is filling with blood from the rest of the body. When the right and left ventricular muscles relax, blood flows from both atria into both ventricles at the same time. The contraction of the atria expels more blood into the ventricular cavities. While the ventricles are filling, the mitral and tricuspid (A-V) valves are open. The same stimulus, originating from the ventricular pacemaker, that excites the right ventricle passes over a specialized network of tissues on the inside of the heart to stimulate the contraction of the left ventricle. As the pressure in the left ventricular cavity builds up, the two leaflets of the mitral valve billow like two sails in the wind to close off the opening between the left atrium and the left ventricle. This prevents blood from regurgitating backward.

At the outlet of the left ventricle, near its top, is the major artery, called the *aorta*, for transporting oxygenated blood to all of the body. At its junction with the left ventricle there is another thin-walled, three-leaflet valve called the *aortic valve*, similar to the pulmonary valve for the right ventricle. While the ventricles are filling this valve is closed. Once the right and left ventricles begin to contract both the aortic and pulmonary valves open. With left ventricular contraction, the pressure in the left ventricle mounts and blood is ejected outward into the arteries to the head, abdomen, legs, arms, and all other regions of the body. After contraction of the left ventricle is over, the pressure begins to fall, and the aortic valve snaps shut, preventing blood under pressure in the aorta from regurgitating back into the left ventricular cavity. In this simple manner, the four-chambered heart provides continuous circulation to the lungs and the entire body.

Blood for the Heart Muscle

The working heart muscle requires a blood supply just like any other muscle in the body. The heart muscle must have oxygen, nutrients, and essential body chemicals, otherwise it cannot properly do its muscular work. It is this critical blood supply to the heart muscle that is directly involved in heart attacks. For this reason, the blood supply to the heart is of particular importance. As the oxygenated blood leaves the left ventricle and enters the aorta, there are two small openings just beyond the aortic valve at the base of the aorta. These are the two openings into the arteries

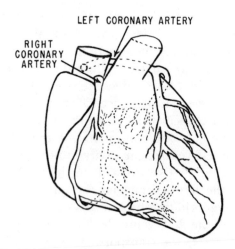

LEFT CORONARY ARTERY

RIGHT CORONARY ARTERY

that supply the heart muscle. One of these extends over the right and back sides of the ventricular muscle mass and is called the *right coronary artery*. The other opening leads into the artery that supplies chiefly the left side, part of the front, and the back of the heart muscle. This is called the *left coronary artery*. These two major arteries are responsible for almost all of the blood that is available for the heart muscle. The left coronary artery soon branches into two major divisions, one of which extends over the front of the ventricular muscle mass and the other of which extends predominantly over the left side and back of the heart. This early division of the left coronary artery sometimes gives rise to the statement that there are three main arteries to the heart.

These arteries are on the outside of the heart muscle and are easily observed if the heart is exposed. Like arteries elsewhere in the body they immediately begin to branch into a larger number of smaller arteries. Some of these also extend over the surface of the heart and others begin to penetrate directly into the heart muscle. The smaller of these arteries become more and more thin-walled to gradually form a spongelike network for the transmission of blood along the heart muscle fibers. The terminal branches of these arteries sometimes interconnect with each other. In the most desirable circumstances, terminal branches of the right coronary artery connect with terminal branches of the left coronary artery. This, in effect, allows an opportunity for a detour of blood from one artery to the other.

The connections between the terminal branches of the right and left coronary arteries really are nature's way of creating a redundancy of the system. If the right coronary artery were to be closed, blood should be able to get through to the heart muscle via the left coronary artery. Unfortunately, these connections are not always open or adequately developed. If they are not, nature's redundancy is lost and the heart muscle is susceptible to any sudden interruption of blood supply caused by blockage of any of the major branches of the coronary arteries. Obstruction of a coronary artery or an inadequate blood supply to part of the heart muscle is the usual cause of a heart attack.

All of the little arterial branches finally connect into small, thin-walled veins. The smaller veins join into larger veins which enter into a single vein emptying into the right atrial reservoir with the rest of the relatively unoxygenated blood.

A Sac for the Heart

The entire four-chambered heart and the origin of its great vessels are enclosed in a saclike membrane called the *pericardial sac*

(sac around the heart). The bottom of the pericardial sac rests on top of the diaphragm. Within the sac is a small amount of straw-colored fluid. Under certain abnormal conditions the sac may become filled with an excessive amount of fluid, causing pressure on the heart itself. Inflammation of this sac, or the external surface of the heart, is called *pericarditis*—meaning inflammation around the heart. Actually, outer portions of the heart muscle are also involved. Although such conditions are painful (often following in the wake of a respiratory infection) the vast majority of them are not usually fatal. Most individuals recover from such episodes without residual ill-effects. At the onset of the illness it often is difficult for the doctor to differentiate pericarditis from a heart atack.

Capillaries, Veins, and Arteries

As the major arteries, pulmonary and aorta, leave the heart, they give off successive branches which in turn give off more branches to provide the network of circulation. Eventually, fine thin-walled structures extend from the arteries past individual muscle fibers and cells. These small, thin-walled structures are called *capillaries*. They are responsible for the circulation at the cellular level. Fluid leaves the blood stream in the capillaries and bathes the individual cells. It then returns to the capillary to maintain the blood volume. The small capillaries finally begin to coalesce, forming larger channels which are small veins. These small veins gradually aggregate into larger veins, all of which eventually empty into the great veins returning blood to the right side of the heart.

The arteries have thicker walls than the veins. Actually, the arteries are composed of several different layers of tissue. The internal layer or lining of the arteries is called the *intima*. Directly beneath the intima are small elastic fibers which are called the *elastic membrane*. External to the elastic membrane is a heavy layer of muscle tissue, interspersed with some elastic elements. Surrounding the muscular layer is a thin, sheathlike external lining. The size of the opening in the artery can be controlled by contracting or relaxing the muscle layer. These tiny muscle fibers are continuously active independent of man's consciousness. The muscle tissue is constantly receiving nerve signals or chemical stimuli which influence its state of contraction or relaxation. In most parts of the body the nervous system has a direct effect upon the muscle layer. Certain nerve fibers, when stimulated, cause the arterial muscle to relax, thereby opening the lumen, or passageway, of the artery, enabling it to accommodate a greater volume of blood. Other nerve fibers, upon appropriate signal, cause the muscle layer to contract, decreasing or closing off the lumen, thus impeding or stopping the flow of blood through this area. A sudden violent contraction of the arterial muscle is called an *arterial spasm*. Some authorities believe that muscle spasms of this type can occur in the coronary artery, causing *coronary spasm*.

The nervous regulation of the arterial muscle enables the body to readjust automatically the amount of blood going to any one portion of the body. If a man is running and needs more blood in his legs, the tiny muscles of the arterial walls relax to permit a greater portion of the blood to be shunted to the working leg muscles. The arterial muscle layer is also responsive to various chemicals created by the body. Some of these chemicals cause the vessels to constrict while others cause them to dilate. For example, when the adrenal gland is stimulated it may release one form of adrenaline which causes constriction of the arteries by muscular contraction or another form of it which causes dilation by relaxation of tiny muscle fibers. Similarly, the physician may use different drugs to produce a direct effect upon the state of the arterial muscle. In the case of shock, drugs may be used to elevate the blood pressure by causing arteriolar constriction or to lower it by causing relaxation of the arterial muscle fibers.

The capillaries are essentially devoid of muscle and represent an almost membrane-like structure. Blood flowing through the capillaries is frequently controlled by a small cuff of tiny muscular tissue just preceding the capillary, which is under the control of various nerve and chemical influences.

Most veins do have a muscular layer, although it is not nearly as thick as that found in the arteries. The arteries are often subjected to very high levels of pressure created by the pumping action of the heart. The veins must accommodate a large volume of blood under relatively low pressure. The movement of blood in the large veins is often facilitated by small valvelike structures, which allow the blood to flow only in one direction. These are found, for example, in the leg veins.

Anatomy of the Killer

There are many ways in which the arteries and veins can be diseased, including inflammation from a variety of disorders. The most important disease of the arteries, however, and the one that causes the vast majority of heart attacks and strokes is caused by the deposition of the fattylike substance *cholesterol* just beneath

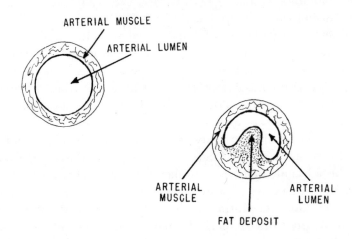

the intima, with its adjacent elastic membrane and heavy muscular layer. As this deposit grows it pushes the intimal lining into the lumen of the vessel, gradually decreasing the size of the opening. If the vessel is large and the deposit is relatively small, there will be no apparent problem. A localized deposit of fatty material, however, may grow to the point of rupturing the intimal lining of the blood vessels—much as rust can flake off from the inner lining of a pipe and occlude its opening. When such an event occurs in the coronary artery it is called a *coronary occlusion*. A blood clot (*thrombosis*) may form at the site of the deposit giving rise to the term *coronary thrombosis*. Blockage of an artery may impair the blood supply to an area of tissue, causing cell death. This process is called an *infarction*. Death of heart muscle (*myocardium*) is called a *myocardial infarction;* death of lung tissue is a *pulmonary infarction;* death of kidney tissue is a *renal infarction,* and so forth.

The deposition of fatty material in the vessel wall is reversible up to a point. To some extent fat is stored in the vessel wall just as it is stored elsewhere in the body when excessive fat is available. During periods when the fat deposits are needed for metabolism they are mobilized from the arteries just as they are mobilized from fat deposits under the skin. If the fat deposit remains for a long period of time, secondary changes may occur. The original soft, pliable, mushylike material gradually hardens. The hard, thick substance is then called a *plaque*. In some of the plaques small deposits of calcium will occur, causing the artery to have a bonelike structure. The gamut of changes associated with fat deposits in the blood vessel wall to the formation of plaques and calcifications is encompassed under the general term *atherosclerosis*, or simply "hardening of the arteries."

Calcification of the muscular layer of the artery can occur without affecting the size of the vessel lumen. This type of rigid hardening of the arteries is not commonly associated with heart attacks or deficient blood supply to a vital organ. It does decrease the natural elasticity of the arteries and influences the blood pressure. Essentially it causes the arteries to become rigid, nonexpansile tubes, whereas in a normal state, the elastic arteries expand and contract in a flexible fashion. When blood is ejected from the heart into the great aorta, the elastic artery readily expands to accommodate a great deal of the blood volume thereby limiting the rise of blood pressure. In older people, when this elasticity is lost the blood pressure rises.

Atherosclerosis may occur in arteries anywhere in the body. If a vital artery is significantly occluded it can affect the function of a tissue normally receiving its blood supply through that vessel. An example of this is seen in older individuals who develop changes in the arteries that severely limit the blood flow to the legs. When such an obstruction exists the individual often can walk only for a short distance before developing fatigue or actual pain in the leg muscles. The pain commonly disappears immediately, when walking is stopped.

Blood Flow to the Brain

In the brain, as in many other areas of the body, nature has provided a redundancy of the system. Basically, the brain is supplied by four major arteries. Two of these enter the skull through the spinal column. These are joined by another pair originating from the carotid arteries that can be felt in the neck on both sides of the voice box. These four arteries connect to form a common arterial ring at the base of the brain. Because of this interconnection, occlusion of one of the four vessels between the heart and the ring may be compensated by blood flow from the remaining vessels. When the atherosclerotic process begins to involve more than one vessel to the brain or when the connections between the different vessels are inadequate, problems of blood flow to the brain occur and may cause a stroke.

Occasionally obstructions to the blood flow to the brain may be found in the major arteries closer to the heart. Some of these may be in the major arteries going up the neck or in other regions coming directly off the great aorta shortly after it leaves the heart. When such defects can be found and are relatively localized, the artery may be opened and cleaned out, much as you would bore out rust from a pipe. Another surgical approach is the arterial bypass operation, using a tube made of a new synthetic material such as Dacron. One end of the tube is connected to the artery below the obstruction and the other end beyond it, bypassing the blockage. Such procedures are particularly advantageous when the obstruction to the brain is located early, before it has caused significant permanent damage. In such instances, a procedure of this sort may prevent the occurrence of a stroke.

At present there is very little that can be done about arterial disease of the brain within the skull once it has occurred. The surgical approach is difficult, if not impossible. Once an area of the brain has been damaged, there are often permanent residual effects. To a limited extent other areas of the brain can be trained to take over functions that have been lost. This essentially is what is accomplished when one retrains an individual to speak who has lost his speaking ability following a stroke. In other instances there is some recovery of brain and nerve function which implies that the tissue was never completely dead but only incapacitated on a temporary basis. Strokes represent essentially the same disease process that causes heart attacks, except that the artery involved supplies the brain instead of the heart muscle.

Filtering the Blood

The circulation to the kidney is unique because of the role this organ plays in filtering out the waste products of metabolism as well as controlling the water balance of the body. The great aorta curves across the top of the chest and descends downward into the abdomen. Branches of this main artery go to each kidney. These are called the *renal arteries*. They divide and enter into small grapelike structures of the kidney which are literally the filtering plant of the kidney itself. Each small artery emerges from a grapelike structure, finally entering into capillaries which collect together into large veins to emerge from the kidney as the *renal vein*. The renal veins enter the great inferior vena cava to drain directly back to the right atrial reservoir.

Not only does the kidney function as a large filtering plant but it also secretes chemical substances or hormones. When there is insufficient blood flow to the kidney these chemical substances cause the blood pressure to rise. This is apparently one of nature's mechanisms designed to insure adequate continued filtration. When all of these mechanisms function in the normal physiological manner they are useful control systems. On the other hand, if the blood supply to the kidney is abnormally interrupted, these events can result in abnormal elevation of blood pressure, or hypertension. Some of those instances where hypertension is caused by abnormal circulation to the kidney can be corrected surgically. This is done in a manner similar to the procedures described for bypassing an obstruction of the blood flow to the brain. Again, a tube made of a synthetic material may be used to bypass an obstruction outside of the kidney, or, if the obstruction is sufficiently localized, the vessel may be opened and the lumen cleaned by boring out the abnormal material. Occasionally some body structure or ligament, externally occluding the blood vessel to the kidney, may be corrected surgically. When the disease of the arteries extends into the internal portion of the kidney there is very little which can be done. A common cause for disease of the kidneys is the silent killer, the atherosclerotic process with the accumulation of fatlike deposits in the wall of the renal artery causing the gradual occlusion of the blood supply to the kidney itself. Interestingly enough, elevation of blood pressure seems to accelerate or increase the deposit of fatty substances in the arterial wall. When this affects the blood vessels to the kidney, it can cause elevation of blood pressure. In such a manner a vicious cycle may be established.

The Chow Line

All organs must have a flow of oxygenated blood through an arterial system. This includes the stomach, intestines, and liver. These organs of the *gastrointestinal tract* are unusually rich with veins, hence it is the venous system that absorbs most of the nutrient materials from the intestinal tract. This complex system of veins joins into larger veins which enter the liver as the *portal vein.* The liver may be regarded as a very large sponge, full of venous blood coming directly from the intestinal tract. The vast majority of blood in the liver is relatively unoxygenated, or venous blood. After the liver has carried out its necessary metabolic functions, the blood leaves the spongelike structure to join the inferior vena cava or the great vein that transports blood from the lower portion of the body back to the right atrium.

Circulation of Lymph

An auxiliary part of the circulation is the *lymphatic system.* Everyone is familiar with the large glands in the neck that swell when the throat is sore and the painful lumps that develop under the arm during a hand infection. These are lymph glands, which generate white blood cells and protective substances to fight off infections. The secretions from them is *lymph,* a clear to milky fluid. A small network of lymph vessels collect the secretions from the lymph glands throughout the body—from the foot to the hand, from the throat to the intestinal tract. The lymph vessels eventually collect into one large vessel called the *thoracic duct.* This large vessel is near the vertebral column in the thorax and empties into the inferior vena cava. Through the thoracic duct the lymphatics connect directly to the venous portion of the circulation. The lymphatic system is vital to the transport of fat from the intestine and to the collection of fat particles that pass through the blood vessel wall. This is discussed more fully in Chapter VI on Food, Fat, and Fate.

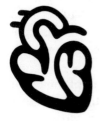

C H A P T E R   I I I

How It Works

WHAT SORT OF reaction do you have when you see blood? Some people faint at the sight of it. To others it often means some form of violence, bravery, or tragedy. It is sometimes linked to guilt, as implied in the old expression, "the blood will be on your hands," or finds its way into the pages of history, as in Churchill's famous phrase, "blood, toil, tears, and sweat." Blood has a deep spiritual meaning, particularly to many primitive people. Blood is essential to life. It was not too many years ago that man learned to transfuse blood from one man to another. To the extent that blood may be considered an organ, blood transfusions were the first successful organ transplants. It is this complex fluid that the heart and vascular system transports throughout the body. It is essential to the function of the circulation as a transport mechanism. When disease of an artery impedes or prevents distribution of this vital fluid to an area of tissue, the tissue dies.

The Magic Fluid

The amount and composition of blood is carefully regulated by a number of complex mechanisms. In the adult male, the total amount of blood in the body is between six and eight liters.* The

* In the metric system, which is commonly used for measurements for medicine, the liter is a little more than a quart; thus the blood volume is approximately two gallons.

total amount of blood (two gallons) is simply called the *blood volume*. The blood volume is actually a suspension of cells and other substances in a fluid. The red blood cells give blood its color. If the red blood cells and white blood cells are allowed to settle, a clearer straw-colored fluid called *plasma* remains. The plasma constitutes approximately fifty-five per cent and the cells forty-five per cent of the total blood volume.

The role of the plasma is of great importance. It is plasma that seeps out of the circulatory system to mix with the fluid that bathes the individual tissue cells. Through this process various elements are transported to and from the cell. Fluid carrying waste products from the tissue cells returns to the blood volume to be carried away for disposition. The actual exchange of gases, nutrients, and waste products at the cellular level is dependent upon the flow of the blood plasma.

Suspended within the plasma are small protein molecules (*albumen, globulin,* and *fibrinogen*). For the most part, these are sufficiently large that they cannot migrate out of the vascular tree. They influence the movement of fluid into and out of the blood stream. If too much fluid leaves the plasma and migrates out to the cellular area, the protein molecules become more densely concentrated and tend to draw fluid back to the circulating blood stream by absorption. At the arterial end of the capillaries, fluid tends to leave the circulation, carrying nutrient elements and oxygen to bathe the tissue cells. The high arterial pressure contributes to this external migration of fluid. Farther along the capillary, near its venous end, the internal pressure is significantly lower. At this point, the plasma proteins act to draw fluid back into the vascular reservoir. This process is based on the simple chemical principle that particles in suspension on one side of a membrane tend to draw fluid through the membrane to dilute their concentration. The plasma proteins thus maintain blood volume by causing fluid to be returned to the venous portion of the circulation, after it has bathed the tissues.

There are many different chemicals in the plasma such as sugar. When a physician draws blood samples from his patient and measures the sugar content of the plasma, he gains information concerning whether or not a patient has diabetes. Usually the chemical composition of the body is determined by chemical analysis of the blood plasma. Measurements of the salt content include sodium, potassium, calcium, chlorides, and other chemicals called the *electrolyte content.*

Just as the blood sugar is one indication of the metabolic action of the body, the functions of various organs can be assessed by the concentration of various chemicals in the plasma. When the kidneys are not functioning properly nitrogenous wastes increase in the plasma. A variety of chemicals provides information on the function of the liver. Several of the fatty substances in the blood are the bases for epidemiological studies that have been done in relationship to heart disease. The best known of these is *blood cholesterol,* which organic chemists call a *solid alcohol.* It is present in large amounts in bile, accounting for the word *cholesterol,* which is derived from Greek, meaning "bile solid." Deposition of this substance in the arterial wall is a major factor in the development of atherosclerosis, or the mushy fat deposit beneath the inner lining of the arteries. Cholesterol is absolutely essential to life. It is found in the brain, the adrenal glands, and almost all cells. Many investigators think that the amount of cholesterol found in the plasma of the circulating blood has a direct bearing upon its abnormal deposition in the arterial walls. For this reason, measuring the blood cholesterol has become a frequent part of annual examinations. Some physicians judge the progress of their patients in terms of diet, medications, and other procedures by evaluating the level of their blood cholesterol.

The amount of various nutrient substances in the blood varies greatly in relation to eating. The different nutrient substances absorbed from the gastrointestinal tract increase their concentration in the plasma immediately. Eating a candy bar, ingesting any form of sugar water or other sugar-containing food causes the blood sugar to increase. Nutrients are transported by the blood stream to the liver, where they undergo chemical action to prepare them for storage in various parts of the body, or for immediate use to meet energy requirements. Within a short period of time, usually two hours, after having eaten a sugar-sweetened substance, the amount of sugar in the plasma will return to the level noted before eating.

The bloodstream contains its own clotting and repair system, consisting of *platelets,* fibrinogen (one of the three types of protein molecules noted before), and various enzymes. When a blood vessel is cut or damaged, a chemical reaction begins which allows the aggregation of sticky protein molecules called fibrin. These coalesce and trap red blood cells within the fibers. This sticky aggregation will stop the bleeding of a small cut or, in the case of an acute heart attack, will occlude the lumen of the artery. When the internal lining, or intima, of the artery is ruptured from the underlying accumulation of fatty deposits, fibrin-like products are laid down and a clot or a thrombosis results. If a specimen of blood is allowed to clot in a test tube the fibrin-like material will entrap the red blood cells and other cellular elements, then gradually contract into a clotted mass. The remaining substance, called *serum*, is even clearer than the usual plasma. Many of the blood chemical analyses, such as the determination of cholesterol and electrolytes, are made from this substance and represent serum values. The actual volume difference between serum and plasma is not great. Certain chemicals, such as citrates, can prevent the clotting mechanism from occurring. These are in common use in blood banks and in situations where unclotted blood must be collected or stored.

Gas in the Blood

The different gases involved in respiration are also dissolved in the plasma. All gases have a certain degree of solubility in fluid, just as sugar has its level of solubility in water. If you add too much sugar to a glass of water the extra sugar will accumulate in the bottom of the glass. The amount of sugar which can be dissolved by the water before the settling occurs is an index of the solubility of sugar in water. In a similar manner, oxygen, carbon dioxide, and nitrogen—the important gases related to respiration—are soluble in fluids. Their solubility is related to temperature and pressure. Oxygen dissolved in water creates a pressure of its own called *oxygen tension*. One may also speak of *carbon dioxide tension* or of *nitrogen tension*. Atmospheric pressure at sea level literally pushes a small quantity of oxygen into solution in water. If the water is then taken to a higher altitude, the amount of pressure forcing oxygen to be dissolved in water is decreased, and a certain amount of oxygen will escape.

At sea level everything is subjected to one atmosphere of pressure, which is 760 mmHg (14.7 pounds per square inch). The accumulation of gaseous pressure, or gas tension, exerted by all the atmospheric gases on a glass of water at sea level would be 760 mmHg. Since room air at sea level contains approximately twenty-one per cent oxygen, the oxygen tension for the oxygen dissolved in the glass of water would be twenty-one per cent of 760 mmHg, or 159.60 mmHg. Under these circumstances, the tension of oxygen in the water is in equilibrium with the atmospheric pressure. If the oxygen tension in the water exceeds that of the oxygen tension in the atmosphere, oxygen will escape from the glass of water. If it is less than the pressure of oxygen in the atmosphere, the glass of water will absorb oxygen. This principle explains how the circulation transports oxygen and carbon dioxide to and from the tissue cells.

Circulating Storage Tanks

The red blood cells may be thought of as storehouses for oxygen or carbon dioxide. Since only a small amount of these gases can be dissolved in the plasma, a means must exist to store larger volumes of the gases in the blood. This is accomplished by the unique characteristics of the red blood cells. The red blood cells play no part in the actual transfer of gases from the blood stream to the various tissues—a function carried on by the fluid leaving and returning to the plasma. The red blood cells are simply specialized storehouses or reservoirs.

Each tiny sphere-shaped red blood cell has within it a chemical substance called *hemoglobin,* with a peculiar ability by virtue of its chemical structure to absorb and carry large quantities of oxygen and carbon dioxide. Many people are familiar with the use of carbon in gas masks because of its ability to absorb large quantities of gas. Although the chemical combinations are different, the principle is the same; a small amount of hemoglobin can carry a reasonably large volume of oxygen. In the metric system this is expressed by stating that one gram of hemoglobin can carry 1.34 ml of oxygen.* As a generalization, it could be said that under sea level conditions one volume of hemoglobin will combine with approximately one and one-half to two volumes of oxygen.

* A milliliter (ml) is one-thousandth of a liter, or a little more than one-thousandth of a quart. Four milliliters is equivalent to one teaspoonful. A liter of water, under standard conditions, weighs 1000 grams or 2.2 pounds. A liter of heavy substances such as mercury, of course, weighs much more, while a liter of light substances, such as a liter of gas, weighs far less.

The hemoglobin molecule contains iron, and it is this fact that relates an iron deficiency to anemia. Insufficient iron stores represent insufficient hemoglobin in the red blood cells, which in turn results in a diminished capacity to carry oxygen. With the help of some very complex chemical reactions, as long as the amount of oxygen dissolved in the plasma (oxygen tension) is relatively high, oxygen will be loaded into the red blood cell for storage in combination with the hemoglobin molecule. As soon as oxygen begins to leave the plasma, causing the oxygen tension to fall, the hemoglobin molecule begins to unload oxygen into the plasma. This tends to maintain the level of oxygen dissolved in the plasma.

Since carbon dioxide is an end product of metabolism, it must be carried away from the cells. Like oxygen it has an affinity for iron, and hence it combines with hemoglobin and is carried back to the lungs by the bloodstream. As the hemoglobin molecule gives up its oxygen, it takes on carbon dioxide. Red blood cells leaving the lungs are full of oxygen, causing the blood to be the bright-red color commonly seen on free bleeding when blood meets air. After the red blood cell releases its oxygen and takes on carbon dioxide, the hemoglobin molecule changes its color and the blood becomes a very dark, dusky color. The color of the blood will depend upon the relative amounts of oxygen and carbon dioxide in the red blood cells. The oxygen-poor blood as seen through the walls of the vein appears blue, and causes a bluish coloration of the veins in the hands and external surface of the body. In the blood that has bathed the heart muscle, almost all of the oxygen is removed. For this reason, if one draws a sample of venous blood from the coronary veins draining the heart muscle, the blood will be very dark, almost black in appearance. If a sufficient amount of unoxygenated blood is circulating through the tissues like the lips, nose, or face, it will impart a bluish discoloration to the tissues, and this is called *cyanosis,* sometimes seen in children born with birth defects. This same bluish discoloration of the skin, however, can occur in normal infants when the blood is slowed or stagnated in the skin during severe crying episodes or breath holding.

The Oxygen Supply Station

In evaluating the function of the heart and circulatory system as a transport mechanism, many calculations related to the transport of oxygen are performed. Oxygen is supplied to the circulatory system by the tiny air sacs (*alveoli*) in the lungs. Each one of these little air sacs comes in direct contact with the capillary blood and only a thin membrane separates the circulating blood from the air space. The mixture of gases in the air sac is slightly different from that in the atmosphere. This is because only a small amount of the air in all of the air sacs is moved in and out with each respiration. The dead space which is the windpipe (*trachea* and *bronchi*), nose, and nasal passages also limits the amount of air actually exchanged. The lungs' function maintains a gas mixture in the air sacs containing thirteen per cent oxygen. The rest of the gases are nitrogen, carbon dioxide, and vaporized water.

Whereas the pressure of oxygen in the atmosphere at sea level is 159.60 mmHg (twenty-one per cent of 760 mmHg), the pressure of oxygen in each air sac is only about 100 mmHg. This can be changed by rapid and deep breathing or momentarily by exhaling as much air as possible from the lungs, then drawing in a complete new supply of air, but these effects of course are transitory.

Transporting the Oxygen

Gas tensions tend to equalize on each side of a membrane. For this reason, the oxygen tension in the blood leaving the air sac of the lung is the same as the oxygen tension in the alveolus, or approximately 100 mmHg. This is exactly the same principle that causes the oxygen tension in a glass of water at sea level to come into equilibrium with the oxygen tension in the room air. The oxygen tension in the blood is directly related to the amount of oxygen dissolved in the plasma, which is much less than the blood is capable of carrying because of the affinity of oxygen for hemoglobin. If all of the hemoglobin in the blood combines with oxygen (at a rate of 1.34 ml of oxygen for each gram of hemoglobin), the amount of oxygen contained in 100 ml of blood (one-tenth liter) would be approximately 19.5 to 20.0 ml of oxygen. This would represent the maximum amount of oxygen that the blood could absorb under room-air conditions and is called its *oxygen capacity*. Actually, the arterial blood almost never carries its total capacity of oxygen; it is like a truck that is not quite loaded. There are a number of factors which contribute to this, the most important one being that a small amount of unoxygenated blood going to the lungs does not come in contact with functioning air sacs and returns from the lungs unoxygenated. The actual amount of oxygen in a sample is known as its *oxygen content*. Under normal circumstances the oxygen content of arterial blood is approximately 19 ml. In order to express the effectiveness of the blood in carrying oxygen, the ratio of the oxygen content to oxygen capacity is expressed as a percentage, called the *oxygen saturation*. The usual saturation for the arterial blood leaving the lungs is ninety-seven per cent, which means that the oxygen content of the arterial blood is ninety-seven per cent of the total oxygen capacity of the blood.

Delivering Oxygen to the Cells

As the blood volume courses down the arterial stream and enters the capillaries, the fluid leaving the capillaries carries with it oxygen under a tension of 100 mmHg. The oxygen-enriched fluid surrounds the membrane of the muscle fibers and specialized cells throughout the body. Within each one of these tiny cells nutrient materials have been burned to create energy for cellular function. In the burning, or metabolism, the oxygen in the cells has been utilized. For this reason, there is less oxygen in the tissue cells than in the fluid coming out of the circulatory system. The amount of gas pressure created by the remaining oxygen dissolved in the cell may be 40 mmHg or less. Immediately, the oxygen dissolved in the fluid will move across the cell membrane to replenish the stores of oxygen in the cell.

The amount of carbon dioxide (CO_2) in the cell builds up as the result of the metabolic process. This CO_2 pressure is greater than that in the external fluid and carbon dioxide moves out of the cell. The fluid bathing the different tissue cells is like a great mixing vat of chemical substances. Its oxygen tension keeps falling because oxygen is being taken up by the cells while its carbon dioxide tension keeps rising because it is leaving the cells. The miles and miles of tiny capillaries emersed in this fluid interact with the tension of gases in all the different tissue spaces. The plasma within the entire capillary bed continues to unload oxygen and pick up carbon dioxide, reaching some degree of equilibrium with the amount of gases in the different tissues. While the oxygen is rapidly being picked up by the individual tissue cells, the amount in the plasma begins to fall, causing the red blood cell reservoirs to

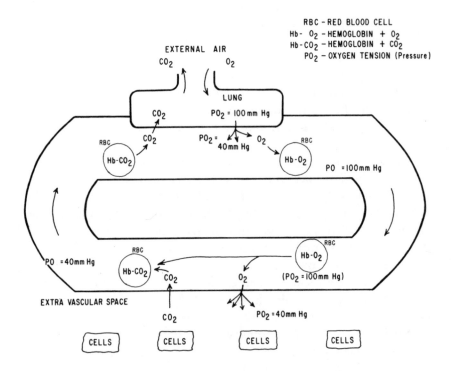

come to the rescue. Immediately chemical reactions cause the hemoglobin to unload its surplus oxygen into the plasma stream. With this unloading, the oxygen content and the oxygen tension of the plasma are maintained. The result of the unloading of oxygen is a sharp decrease in the oxygen content of the circulating blood. This, of course, changes the ratio of oxygen content to oxygen capacity so the oxygen saturation decreases and the blood is said to be *unsaturated*.

While this process is occurring at different degrees throughout the body, the continuously moving blood stream gradually propels its way back to the right heart. In the right atrial reservoir there is a mixing of all of the blood that has given up oxygen to different parts of the body. Under normal resting circumstances the fast-moving stream of blood throughout the tissues does not give up all of its oxygen. The mixed venous blood in the right atrial chamber usually still contains about 14 ml of oxygen in each 100 ml unit. The circulating red blood cells and plasma leave the lungs fully loaded with oxygen, then make the trip around the body and return to the heart still containing about seventy per cent of their oxygen load. This residual oxygen is another one of nature's redundant mechanisms. It is a reserve supply of oxygen that can be used during periods of stress or unexpected needs. The oxygen content of the venous blood coming back from the legs, kidneys, and upper portions of the body, under resting circumstances remains fairly high. *The sole exception, and a very important one indeed, is the venous blood returning from the heart muscle. The heart is the only place in the body where almost all of the oxygen is extracted from its blood supply under resting circumstances.* Even while an individual is sitting quietly in a chair or lying in bed, the oxygen saturation of the blood coming back from the heart muscle is only about twenty-five per cent, with an oxygen content of 4 or 5 ml. This is about as much oxygen as can be extracted from the circulating bloodstream. The coronary blood flow literally gives up under resting conditions about as much oxygen as can be extracted from the circulating blood. Clearly, *there is only one way that more oxygen can be provided for increased work of the heart and that is by increasing the coronary blood flow.* Since no more oxygen can be extracted from each unit of blood, the alternative is to increase the number of units of blood bathing the heart muscle.

Oxygen Consumption and How Much the Heart Pumps

The metabolic actions of the different cells of the body require oxygen. The amount of oxygen used by the body can be measured by simple techniques. The oxygen consumption of the body has a direct bearing upon the work of the circulation, since it is the circulating blood that must transport the oxygen to be consumed. Utilizing this principle, a method was devised to determine how much blood the heart actually pumped in any given minute.

The principle is really very simple. If each 100 ml unit of blood leaving the lungs contains 19 ml of oxygen and after it has unloaded a portion of this oxygen to the tissues, it returns to the heart with 14 ml of oxygen—one knows that each 100 ml unit of blood delivers 5 ml of oxygen to the body. By measuring the oxygen consumed through the lungs during this period of time, if it is determined that the individual has consumed a total of 250 ml of oxygen, it is obvious that it requires fifty units of blood to deliver the oxygen to the tissues. Since each unit of blood that gives up 5 ml of oxygen represents 100 ml, it is clear that fifty units represent 5000 ml or five liters. From such calculations it has been determined that in the resting adult the heart pumps an average of five liters (over five quarts) of blood a minute. This is called the *cardiac output*. There may be marked variation from moment to moment and the heart can increase its pumping ability (cardiac output) manyfold when required to do so.

Pumping Action of One Beat

Determining the cardiac output by measuring the oxygen consumption is as simple as determining how many trucks are required to move a given number of bushels of wheat per hour. In breaking down the functions of the heart, it is sometimes desirable to know how much blood is pumped by the heart each time it beats. Each contraction of the heart to produce its pumping effect is called a stroke, and the volume that is pumped with each contraction is called the *stroke volume*. If you know that the heart pumps five liters of blood a minute and if the heart beats sixty-six times a minute, it is a simple matter to divide the cardiac output by the heart rate to obtain a figure of 75 ml (about one-third cup) —the average amount of blood pumped by each beat of the heart. Under normal resting conditions the ventricles only eject about half of the blood they contain. The volume of the left ventricle may easily be as much as 150 ml in a young man in good physical condition, though only half of this amount, or 75 ml, is ejected with each stroke. The residual volume of blood in the left ventricle is one more example of nature's redundancy. It is an additional capacity which the heart can call upon when it needs to increase the amount of blood it pumps per minute.

What Causes Your Blood Pressure

When the pressure inside the ventricular chamber equals or slightly exceeds the pressure in the large aorta, the aortic valves open and blood rushes out into the aorta. The 75 ml of blood ejected into the already filled aorta increases the pressure within the artery. The peak of this pressure is called the *systolic pressure*. This is the high reading taken during a normal physical examination. As the doctor examines his patient he places a cuff around the upper part of the arm and listens through a stethoscope for heart sounds in the arteries below the cuff. The pressure in the cuff is inflated to the point that it occludes the underlying artery so that blood stops at the cuff. By gradually releasing the pressure in the cuff, a point is reached where the pressure in the artery equals the external occlusion pressure of the constricting cuff. At this point, blood begins to flow through the arteries permitting heart sounds to be heard by the doctor through his stethoscope. This point is taken to be equivalent to the systolic pressure within the artery. Its value varies greatly, but in young men it is commonly between 110 and 135 mmHg. The systolic pressure represents the force exerted by the heart muscle to expel blood through the artery.

The volume of blood pumped by the heart at a given level of pressure is the effective work of the heart. Imagine for a moment that the aorta were severed and there was no resistance to the flow of the blood out of the heart each time it pumped. In such a case the amount of pressure required to pump 75 ml of blood each time would be very small, consequently the effective work the heart muscle would have to do would be minimal. On the other hand, if you took a string and tied it firmly around the aorta, gradually reducing its size, it would offer an obstruction to the outflow of blood. The heart would have to work much harder to pump the blood past the obstruction. This would cause a rise in pressure between the heart and the obstruction or an increase in the effective work of the heart muscle.

Although the aorta commonly does not have such an obstruction around it, all the small terminal arteries, plus the aorta filled with blood, do offer resistance to the addition of more blood to the system. This resistance to the flow of blood through the arterial tree (*peripheral resistance*) and the amount of blood pumped by the heart are the essential determinants of blood pressure. The relationship between the amount of blood pumped (blood flow or cardiac output), the resistance offered to the blood flow (peripheral resistance), and the blood pressure is expressed as an equation:

$$\text{blood pressure} = \frac{\text{cardiac output}}{\text{peripheral resistance}}$$

This relationship is important in understanding the function of the heart. If the resistance offered by the vascular tree is not altered but the amount of blood that the heart must pump is increased, the blood pressure will rise—increasing the work of the heart. The work of the heart can also be decreased by decreasing the peripheral resistance. This is done by certain drugs which can cause relaxation of the muscles in the small arteries or through nerve reflex mechanisms.

The amount of blood flow out of the heart into the arteries rises rapidly during contraction of the heart. Gradually the pressure in the aorta and the left ventricle begins to equalize. Finally, ventricular contraction is no longer sustained and relaxation begins, the pressure in the left ventricular cavity falling below the pressure in the aorta. At this point the aortic valve closes. A large amount of the 75 ml of blood ejected into the aorta causes tensing of the aorta and major arteries. As this volume of blood begins to drain off into the small arteries and capillaries the pressure in the main arteries falls. The drop in pressure continues until the next ventricular contraction begins. The lowest point in this fall is called the *diastolic pressure,* which is also recorded by the doctor on routine physical examination. The blood pressure then is recorded as a fraction, expressing the value of the systolic pressure over that of the diastolic pressure (the highest pressure over the lowest pressure). A normal diastolic pressure may be 76 mmHg. A normal blood-pressure reading could be 130/76 mmHg.

The diastolic pressure may be influenced by many factors. As the heart rate increases there is less time between each successive heartbeat, causing the diastolic pressure to rise. This is true as long as the amount of blood pumped by the heart is maintained. If the smaller arteries offer appreciable obstruction to the runoff of blood into the capillary system, the diastolic pressure will remain high. Drugs or disease conditions which tend to increase the contraction of the muscles in the arteries tend to elevate both the systolic and diastolic pressure.

The difference between systolic and diastolic pressure is the *pulse pressure.* In the illustration given, the difference between 130 mmHg and 76 mmHg would be the pulse pressure, or 54 mmHg. The pulse pressure is significantly influenced by the stroke volume of the heart. As the amount of blood pumped by each heartbeat is increased, the systolic pressure rises and the pulse pressure rises. The variation of pressure in the circulatory system, called the *pulsatile flow,* give it its pulsatile characteristic (and the pulse at the wrist).

The higher levels of pressure created by systole cause blood to flow to the more distal portions of the body under normal circumstances. A constant pressure, halfway between the systolic and diastolic levels might on the surface appear to be effective, but the truth is that only the peak pressure levels can provide adequate circulation in the regions furthest from the heart. This is comparable to the limitations imposed by the constant pressure in the plumbing system of a small city. The individuals who live at the outskirts of the city often don't have enough water pressure for their plumbing facilities, particularly in the summer months when a lot of the water is being utilized for lawn care and other purposes. Intermittent peaking of blood pressure caused by pulsatile flow insures that all of the tissues will obtain an adequate blood supply. It also protects the blood vessels against the sustained high level of pressure that would otherwise be necessary to accomplish this purpose.

Much interest has centered around the characteristics of the pulsatile flow with the advent of open-heart surgery and the possibilities of using an artificial heart. The various machines that are used to replace the pumping action of the heart during the operation must provide an adequate circulation for the body tissues on an interim basis. The question of whether these devices are satisfactory when producing a continuous pressure or whether they should provide a pulsatile flow like the normal heart remains a point of discussion.

Why the Arteries to the Lungs Escape the Killer

The systolic and diastolic pressure in the aorta and the major arteries to the body are much higher than the levels encountered in the pulmonary circulation. The pulmonary artery rapidly branches out into large numbers of smaller arteries, and finally into tiny capillaries that go to all the different air sacs of the lungs. This great vascular bed offers very little resistance to the flow of blood. It is able to accommodate a very large blood volume without significantly stretching the network of vessels. For this reason a normal blood pressure in the pulmonary artery may be 35/15 mmHg.

The importance of pressure to the development of atherosclerosis is well demonstrated by the difference in the arteries to the lungs as compared to those of the rest of the body and heart. The pulmonary artery and its branches, in the absence of disease of the lungs or other diseases associated with increased pressure within the pulmonary artery, seldom presents any significant evidence of abnormal deposits of cholesterol or atheromatous degeneration. This is an important observation, since all other factors, including diet, physical activity, heredity, sex, and stress, obviously must be the same in a given individual. This strongly suggests that the low pressure in the pulmonary artery protects it from atherosclerosis. The walls of the pulmonary arteries are also less thick.

The Long Way Home

Like any other fluid, blood flows from a high pressure area to a low pressure area just as water runs downhill. Beyond the capillaries and entering into the venous circulation, these channels are very large and can accommodate large amounts of blood. The pressure within the venous reservoir, accordingly, is very low. The venous pressure in the leg of a person lying down may be only 14 mmHg. The pressure drops even further in the great veins to the heart. During inspiration, as the chest expands, a negative pressure is created within the thorax, which is responsible for expansion of the lungs. This negative pressure is transmitted to the venous system causing the pressure in the great right atrial reservoir to fall below sea level atmospheric pressure. It is the difference in pressure between the arterial and the venous systems that causes oxygenated blood from the left side of the heart to flow to the venous reservoir.

As long as pressure in the great veins and right atrial reservoir is normal the circulation does not significantly influence the size of the liver and other organs that are essentially specialized appendages of the venous reservoir. If the venous pressure rises, however, the liver may become distended and painful. The pressure in the venous system may rise when the right heart begins to fail. In such instances, an individual seated upright may have enlarged or distended neck veins. You can gain an idea of the amount of pressure in your veins by a very simple procedure. While you are seated upright, hold the hand level with the waist. You can see the distended veins on the back of the hand. Now as the hand is raised well above the heart, the veins collapse. This should occur by the time the hand reaches the level of the neck. If the veins remain distended this suggests that the venous pressure is abnormally high. Of course, in carrying out such a test there must not be any constriction about the arm such as a tight watchband or bracelet.

Where the Blood Goes

A normal individual lying down has a cardiac output of five liters per minute. The caliber of the various arteries is adjusted to control the distribution of the blood flow. The amount of blood pumped by the heart is distributed as follows:

	Per cent
Heart	5
Head	15
Thoracic cage	3
Liver and accessory circulation	30
Kidneys	25
Legs and arms	22

Over half, or fifty-five per cent, of the blood pumped by the heart goes to the organs of the abdomen while the muscles are resting and an individual is lying down.

Although it is an extraordinary organ, constructed in such a way as to provide four chambers for the collection of blood, *the heart is basically a muscle.* The heartbeat represents simple muscle contractions. Each contraction of the heart muscle to pump blood represents cardiac work. Like all other tissues, the working heart must have nutrient substances: proteins, fats, carbohydrates, essential amino acids, and vitamins. The individual heart-muscle fibers must have oxygen to metabolize these substances. The oxygen to the heart muscle is supplied by the blood flow through the coronary arteries. Inadequate oxygen for the heart muscle limits the work of the heart, or may cause a heart attack. The non-beating, resting heart muscle, like any other resting muscle, such as a relaxed leg muscle, requires a certain amount of oxygen to maintain its own normal function. This is the *basal metabolism* of the heart muscle, or the oxygen requirements of the non-contracting muscle fibers. The non-beating basal state for the heart muscle doesn't occur under normal circumstances during life. Studies have been carried out by stopping the beating of an animal's heart and measuring the oxygen consumption of the resting heart muscle.

In certain conditions that increase the general metabolism of the body, one can expect an increased oxygen requirement for the resting heart muscle. An individual with an overactive thyroid is a good example. Not only does an overactive thyroid increase the oxygen requirements for the body as a whole, but specifically it also increases the basic oxygen requirement of the resting heart muscle. This increased demand for oxygen increases the need for coronary blood flow.

A second requirement for increased oxygen to the working heart is related to the elasticity of the heart itself. Each muscle fiber may be considered somewhat like the coil of a bed spring, requiring force to compress it. Each contraction and expansion of the heart involves overcoming a certain amount of stiffness of the muscle spring. This is true of other muscles of the body. If the biceps muscle is contracted rapidly, a lot of the energy which is required—and the oxygen that must be supplied to the contracting muscle—is used in overcoming the internal resistance of the muscle itself. The amount of work required for each contraction of the heart muscle is minimized, if the muscle is pliable and stretches easily. A thick, heavy heart muscle requires more work to overcome its own lack of elasticity with each contraction than a normal heart with thinner walls. In certain disease states there is thickening of the membrane on the inner surface of the heart muscle chamber. This thick, tendonous tissue must be stretched and compressed with each cardiac contraction, increasing the work of the heart. The work of the heart which is dependent upon its own elasticity is referred to as the internal work of the heart. Clearly, the fewer heartbeats, the less internal work required. This is one factor related to the decreased efficiency of the rapidly beating heart. Each time the heart beats it must overcome its own lack of elasticity. Obviously one hundred beats per minute means that this task must be accomplished one hundred times. A heart which pumps the same amount of blood by contracting fifty times per minute is more efficient.

In addition to the oxygen requirements for the fundamental basal metabolism of the heart muscle and the internal work of the heart, there are oxygen and nutritional requirements to carry out the effective work of the heart—its actual pumping of blood at a given pressure. Diseases of the valves or abnormal connections between the chambers of the heart or external vessels all affect the efficiency of the heart in terms of its ability to pump blood. Although there are a number of factors determining the oxygen and nutrition requirements of the heart, the most important ones appear to be the basal metabolism of the heart, the heart rate, and the systolic blood pressure. The sustained pressure required to eject blood represents the force of contraction of the heart muscle; this is closely related to the amount of work the heart must do. The total work of the heart, its oxygen and nutrient requirements, can be changed by altering the basic metabolism of the heart muscle; by changing the internal work (for example, influencing heart rate) ; by changing the systolic blood pressure or strength of contraction of the ventricular muscle mass; or by changing the amount of blood that must be pumped.

Because the heart is frequently called upon to supply large amounts of energy, with little or no preparation, nature has stored within the heart muscle a number of complex chemical compounds which are energy-rich sources. One of these chemical substances is called *creatinine phosphate*. These substances can undergo chemical degradation and liberate energy in the absence of additional oxygen. The released energy can be used by the heart muscle for contraction. These substances must be gradually restored as soon as the work requirement is over. These and other unknown factors allow the heart muscle, as other muscles in the body, to accumulate an *oxygen debt*. The biological marvel is that the muscles can run out of adequate oxygen and continue to function, just as if one were to run out of gasoline and still be able to drive his automobile: This oxygen must be replaced. The ability to borrow energy, so to speak, is called *oxygen debt*. There is a limit to the amount of oxygen debt any one individual can sustain. This limit is related to the health of the heart muscle and to the character or amount of chemical and nutrient stores containing high-energy compounds within the muscle cells.

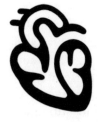

C H A P T E R   I V

Rhythms and Sounds
of the Heart

THE PUMPING ACTION of the heart is normally accomplished in a
synchronized, rhythmic manner. Sometimes the heart beats fast like
a finely tuned engine racing at top speed, or it may beat slowly,
seemingly without effort. The opening and closing of the heart
valves accompanied by the movement of the circulating blood
create the sounds of the heart. The smooth integration of the
heart's pumping action is accomplished by the specialized pacemakers inside the heart and the network of specialized conducting
tissue. The pumping action of the heart results from the inter-
action of electrical stimulation and mechanical response.

What Your Heart Tracing Reveals

A part of every complete heart examination includes a heart
tracing, or *electrocardiogram*. Such an examination can tell the
doctor a great deal about the function of the heart. It gives a
permanent record of the heart rate and tells him which parts of
the heart are stimulated first. The heart tracing gives clues to the
presence of damaged heart muscle or areas of heart muscle that are
not getting sufficient blood supply. The electrocardiogram pinpoints
the presence of a heart attack in a large number of cases and gives the
physician some knowledge concerning its location—whether it is in
the front, back, top, or bottom of the left ventricle. Other changes in

the characteristics of the tracing tell him when the heart muscle undergoes healing. Frequently there is a residual change in the electrical tracing after a heart attack that enables the doctor to know such an attack occurred.

Heart tracings are useful in following the course of different drugs that a patient may be receiving. *Digitalis,* a drug given for heart failure, may cause alterations in the heart tracings and such records help the doctor in determining whether the patient is getting too much or too little medicine. The electrocardiogram even provides information concerning the *electrolytes,* or salt substances in the body. The characteristics of the tracing begin to undergo changes when there is not enough of the salty potassium. If there is too much salty potassium, other changes may occur.

The electrocardiogram provides information concerning the size of the heart and its chambers. Changes develop in the electrocardiogram as the left ventricle enlarges in an individual with high blood pressure. Characteristic changes of the tracing identify conditions in which the right ventricular muscle mass is enlarged. Even enlargement of the large atrial reservoirs causes changes in the electrocardiogram.

Although the physician may obtain clues from the electrocardiogram concerning the state of the heart muscle, the electrical tracing does not provide information by itself concerning the contractural strength of the heart muscle. The mechanical action of the heart must be judged by other means related to heart sounds, blood pressure, and cardiac output.

A Sea Around a Magnet

The ability of the heart to create an electrical signal is one of nature's marvels. The body fluids in and out of the cells for the entire body contain a large amount of electrolytes. Outside the cells the chief salty substance is common table salt, or *sodium chloride.* The amount of salt in the extracellular water is about the same concentration as the salt in sea water. Many scientists link this relationship to the evolutionary theory that mammalian life evolved from creatures of the sea. Inside the cell there is an equal amount of salty substance but the principal salt in this instance is potassium chloride. The electrolytes in the water make the body a good electrical conductor. Any form of electrical activity generated within the body quickly sets up an electrical field throughout the body. The generator for the largest continuous electrical voltage in the body is the heart muscle. Other muscles also create electrical activity when they are stimulated, but under the usual circumstances of a heart examination these muscles are relatively quiet.

The electrical activity of the heart muscle is generated by migration of electrolytes across the cell membranes of the muscle fibers—the migration of potassium and to a lesser extent sodium. These small, charged salt particles change the electrical state of the individual muscle fibers. The electrical result of this change is to cause the heart to act like an electrical generator. It may be thought of at any one moment during its activity as a large magnet. One part of the heart may be considered as the negative pole of the magnet and the other part of the heart muscle, in a different electrical state, may be considered as the positive pole of the magnet. These two poles then represent a dipole and generate a field around it, much like the magnetic field that can be demonstrated around a magnet. During activation of the heart, at any one instant, a large portion of the body can be identified as being the negative part of the electrical field and another portion of the body can be identified as the positive part of the field. When the technician places the electrodes on the arms and legs and across the chest, these electrodes are really used to determine location and strength of the electrical field of the body. This, in turn, depends upon the action of the heart as an electrical generator.

One of the earliest theoretical concepts of the electrocardiogram was advanced by the brilliant Dutch scientist Willem Einthoven. He considered the electrical activity of the heart as being represented by a single dipole, or a single magnet, and the body as a large volume conductor that transmits the electrical field equally throughout its dimensions, as if the heart were a magnet at the center of a large tank of sea water. Using this simple assumption, he was able to work out a number of important concepts related to the electrical activity of the heart. These have stood the test of time and still are used by heart specialists today.

The Heart Has a Spark Plug

The onset of electrical activity is started by the small pacemaker for the right atrial reservoir. This small pacemaker, or spark plug, really lights the fire for excitation. The adjoining muscle fibers in the atria undergo a change related to the migration of electrolytes into and out of the cell. When this change occurs the muscle fiber is said to be excited, which means it is stimulated to the state that leads to its contraction. The cardiac muscle fiber has the property of being able to transmit this stimulus. The stimulus spreads outward across the rest of the atrial muscle fibers much the same way that rings spread out around a pebble dropped into a pool of water. There is, of necessity, a boundary between the tissue which has been excited, and that which has not yet undergone a change. It is this boundary that divides the negative and positive centers of the electrical field, or electrical activity of the heart. The boundary is gradually pushed outward over all of the atrial muscle fibers, both right and left. The electrical field which is generated is picked up by the electrodes for the electrocardiogram and measured as voltage. The first little blip of the electrocardiogram in the normal heart cycle represents the stimulation of the right and then the left atria. This activity, registered on the tracing as a single hump, is called the *P wave*.

There is a pause as the excitation process reaches the pacemaker for the ventricles. Then the impulse spreads slowly through the specialized conducting tissue of the pacemaker for the ventricle, then down into the inner surfaces of both the right and left ventricular muscle. Here, tiny fibers from the specialized conducting tissue are inserted directly into the muscular wall throughout the

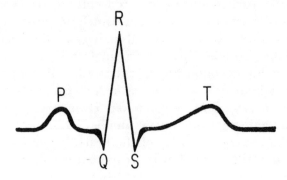

heart muscle chamber. Almost instantaneously, stimulation of all the inner surfaces of the right and left ventricle begins. The stimulation proceeds from inside the heart outward. At each instant these two conical-shaped areas of stimulation moving from the inside out continue to create the effect of a negative and positive field. Following in alphabetical succession, the complex, or series, of spikes that are caused by the electrical excitation of the heart muscle is called the *QRS complex*. If there is dead muscle tissue, or a change in the way in which the wave of stimulation spreads from the inside out over the ventricles, it will alter the shape of this complex in a characteristic manner. This is how damage to the heart muscle, such as that created by heart attacks, and sometimes by inflammatory disorders or other disease, can demonstrate its presence in the electrocardiogram.

Once the heart muscle has been completely excited and contraction ensues, it must be restored to its previous state. This restoration is called *recovery*. When it occurs it again creates an electrical surge or impulse. The surge over the ventricles forms a distinct wave on the heart tracing called the *T wave*. It is this wave that is frequently altered when there is disease of the coronary arteries, when the heart muscle is enlarged, during inflammation, and throughout the entire gamut of heart diseases. It is also changed by a lot of common, everyday facets of life, particularly excitement, anxiety, changes in body position, and recent meals.

What the Doctor Hears

From all of these relatively simple component parts it is possible to put together the sequence of the action of the heart. The resting, dilated phase of the heart, as noted earlier, is called *diastole*. With both the right and left ventricles relaxed, blood pours through the open valves between the ventricles and the atria. This blood is returning to the right atrium through the great veins and to the left atrium from the veins of the lungs to fill the relaxed ventricles.

The rate of activity for the atrial pacemaker (sino-atrial node) is controlled by external nerve influences. On the proper signal the activity of the pacemaker can be increased or decreased. When the pacemaker fires it stimulates the atrial muscle fibers. The impulse sweeps across the atria and down to the pacemaker for the ventricles, and there the impulse pauses. During this pause, the stimulated atrial muscle fibers contract to force more blood collected in the atrial chambers into the dilated and relaxed ventricles.

The ventricles obtain their maximum size at the completion of atrial contraction. Each ventricle may contain as much as 150 ml of blood in the well-conditioned adult male. The stimulation impulse passes through the pacemaker for the ventricles, stimulates the ventricles, and the ventricular muscle mass begins to contract. The apex of the ventricle begins to lift upward toward the top of the heart. As this occurs the large mitral valve between the left atrium and the left ventricle snaps shut. The vibration of its closing is the major component of the first heart sound. Almost simultaneously the three-cusp valve between the right atrium and the right ventricle also snaps shut. The sound of the closure of these two valves constitutes the *first heart sound*. It is heard by the physician just preceding the ejection of blood by the heart's pumping action.

The small valves that guard the outlet to the aorta and pulmonary artery open almost immediately after closure of the two main valves between the upper and lower chambers of the heart. The pressure in the ventricles is greater than the pressure in the great arteries, causing ejection of the cardiac output to begin. Approximately 75 ml of blood are ejected by both the right and left ventricles into their respective main arteries. This starts the arterial pulse and is responsible for the pulse that may be felt at the wrist or in the temple area and other external parts of the body. This period of contraction of the ventricles and ejection of blood into the arterial tree is known as systole.

Once the progressive contraction of the ventricle stops and relaxation begins, the pressure in the right and left ventricular cavity falls sharply. When this occurs, first the aortic valve snaps shut, then almost immediately the pulmonary valve snaps shut—preventing regurgitation of blood into the heart. The closure of these two valves creates another sound called the *second heart sound*. The combination of the first and second heart sounds are the major tones which the doctor hears when he is listening to a normal heart, and they constitute the lub-dub—lub-dub—lub-dub characteristics of the heartbeat.

Shortly after closure of the pulmonary and aortic valves, the falling pressure in the ventricular cavities results in opening of the great valves between the atrial chambers and the ventricular chambers of the heart (A-V valves, or tricuspid and mitral valves). The valves between the atria and ventricles are normally closed during the entire time the ventricles are contracting, or said to be in systole (that period between the first and second heart sounds). This permits the right and the left atrial reservoirs to be filling with blood while the ventricles are contracting. As soon as the A-V valves between the atria and ventricles open the blood which has been accumulated in the atria during ventricular systole dumps into the expanding ventricular cavities. Thus, in a general sense, the right and left atrial reservoirs are filling while the ventricular chambers are emptying by forceful contraction.

What Are Heart Murmurs?

When an abnormal sound is made by the heart, other than the characteristic lub-dub—lub-dub—lub-dub, such sounds are known as heart murmurs. Actually, they are vibrations set up by eddy currents of the flowing blood. Anyone who has ever squeezed on a garden hose while watering the lawn has felt the vibrations caused by the external compression of the hose. Similar vibrations are set up in the vessels and in the heart, and when heard through the stethoscope they are called murmurs. Most heart murmurs are classified by when they occur in the cardiac cycle. To illustrate, a common murmur is caused by incomplete closure of the two-leaflet mitral valve that closes off the left atrium from the left ventricle. As the ventricles begin to contract, the valve snaps shut; if an opening remains, the increased pressure in the left ventricle squirts blood backward into the left atrium, the squirting of blood backward in this fashion creating eddy currents that cause vibrations. Since this occurs during the time that the ventricles are contracting or during ventricular systole, it is called a *systolic murmur*. This alters the heart sounds to lub-*SWISH*-dub—lub-*SWISH*-dub—lub-*SWISH*-dub—.

Incomplete closure of the aortic valve between the great aorta and the left ventricle can permit abnormal blood flow in a similar fashion. The three cusps of the aortic valve come into apposition and close when the ventricles have ceased contraction and begin to dilate for their diastolic phase. If there is a hole or a leak in the valve, the blood under high pressure in the aorta will be squirted back into the relaxing left ventricle. Blood squirting back during this period of time sets up eddy currents and vibrations in the heart which are audible with a stethoscope. Since they occur during the time the ventricular muscle is relaxing or entering into diastole, these are *diastolic murmurs.* The murmur appears in the heart sounds as lub-dub-*SWISH*—lub-dub-*SWISH*—lub-dub-*SWISH*—.

The systolic murmur, caused by incomplete closure of the mitral valve, and the diastolic murmur, caused by the incomplete closure of the aortic valve, are both defects which can occur secondary to rheumatic heart disease. The heart's ability to function as a pump is compromised when such abnormalities are severe. When nature's compensatory mechanisms are exhausted these valves may be replaced by new mechanical valves that have been developed in recent years.

Some murmurs are caused by the rapid ejection of blood squirted outward into the aorta when the left ventricle contracts, setting up vibrations in the aorta. These sounds, occurring during ventricular ejection or systole, also represent systolic murmurs. Some of these are not clinically significant. This is particularly true of systolic murmurs during or immediately after exertion or during excitement. Murmurs of this type may also occur in childhood and in a variety of conditions not related to heart disease, such as anemia. Murmurs that are created on this basis are frequently called *functional or physiological murmurs,* in an attempt to identify them as unrelated to disease of the heart.

The doctor is often faced with the dilemma of trying to decide whether a heart murmur which he has heard when he is examining a child is a functional murmur of childhood or whether it represents heart disease. Often the doctor waits patiently, and the parents somewhat anxiously, to see whether the abnormal sound or murmur persists or disappears as a child grows older. To the satisfaction of the doctor and parents alike, the murmur may disappear and the child grow into a normal, healthy adult with no evidence of abnormality of the heart.

Crazy Rhythm

Many individuals have had the sensation of their heart "skipping a beat." Some describe it as a feeling that their heart turned over in their chest or that an extra-forceful beat of their heart occurred. Others think their heart merely missed a beat. Some individuals note their heart beating rapidly in their chest, and seek advice from their doctor concerning this sensation. Almost all of these events are related to the electrical stimulating action of the heart or its rhythm mechanisms. Some of these are innocuous and do not represent any form of heart disease. Some may go unnoted by the individual. Almost everyone has an occasional abnormal beat of his heart. A lesser number of individuals are aware of these irregularities. In a still smaller number of people, these irregularities are of considerable importance and represent heart disease.

Breathing Irregularity of the Heart

A simple and innocuous variation in heart rate is that associated with breathing. Many parents become alarmed when they note a marked fluctuation in the rate of their child's heartbeat. A careful observation will often demonstrate that this is associated with the respiratory cycle. As the breath is drawn in, the heart rate speeds up—then as the chest reaches full expansion and during the expiratory phase, the heart rate slows. The heartbeat may appear to be irregular when this difference in heart rate between inspiration and expiration is large. The change in heart rate associated with breathing is called *sinus arrhythmia*. It has no importance as far as heart disease is concerned. It is seen characteristically in children and young adults. It disappears often during the adult life only to be noted again in elderly individuals.

What Happens When Your Heart Skips a Beat?

The cause of the skipped beats or simple palpitations that bother some people is frequently an early contraction of the heart. The normal filling period of the heart is interrupted by a premature electrical stimulation of the heart muscle, causing the heart to contract prematurely. The amount of blood ejected by the premature beat may be relatively small, far below the 75 ml stroke volume used earlier as an example. Immediately after the early beat there is a long pause when the heart is relaxed or dilated. This long period allows the heart to fill to greater capacity than it does during normal beats. The first heartbeat after the pause results in the ejection of a much larger volume of blood. This unusually large amount of blood ejected into the aorta causes a large pulsation which may attract the individual's attention. It is not a pain but an unusually strong beat which calls the individual's attention to the irregularity.

Premature beats are sometimes called *extrasystoles.* Regardless of their name the effect is the same. The premature contractions are caused by additional pacemakers in the heart. Nature has provided a large number of auxiliary pacemakers, perhaps in an effort to increase the redundancy of the electrical system for the heart. Some of these extra pacemakers are scattered throughout the atria, others are scattered in the ventricular muscle mass. One of these extra pacemakers may fire out of turn if the sino-atrial node, or normal atrial pacemaker, fails to fire rapidly enough—thereby creating a premature contraction. If the auxiliary pacemaker that fires is in the atria it causes an *atrial premature contraction.* If the pacemaker is in or near the normal pacemaker for the ventricle (A-V node) it may be called a *nodal premature contraction.* A pacemaker in the ventricle may cause a *ventricular premature contraction.*

Attacks of Rapid Heart Action

Sometimes the auxiliary pacemakers may be activated to discharge more rapidly than the normal atrial pacemaker. An auxiliary pacemaker that is able to sustain its action at a more rapid pace than the normal atrial pacemaker will take over the role of stimulating the heart. Such rapid heart action is called an *atrial tachycardia,* if the auxiliary pacemaker is in the atria. This is a frequent cause of palpitation and discomfort that sends patients to see the doctor. An auxiliary pacemaker in the ventricle, that takes over the beating of the heart at a rapid rate, causes *ventricular tachycardia,* which is far less common than atrial tachycardia.

The Twitching Atria

Occasionally, more than one pacemaker may be active in taking over the rhythm of the heart. Most doctors consider that several pacemakers are active in the atria to cause a form of abnormal beating of the heart called *atrial fibrillation.* The active atrial pacemakers stimulate the atria to beat at a very rapid rate, often as fast as five hundred beats a minute. When this occurs the atria literally twitch. Different segments of the atria make small contractions at irregular intervals. Fortunately, only a small number of these impulses can be transmitted by the ventricular pacemaker to stimulate the ventricular muscle mass. As a result the ventricles contract at a much slower rate and, under ideal circumstances, can maintain an adequate cardiac output. Effective atrial contraction is lost in the presence of atrial fibrillation, and the ventricles do not receive the last contribution of blood normally provided by atrial contraction. This, in turn, usually results in a decrease in stroke volume—in the amount of blood pumped with each heart-beat—limiting the amount of blood pumped by the heart. There may not be sufficient time to fill the ventricular cavities before each succeeding contraction, if the ventricles are beating very rapidly in response to any of the abnormalities in rhythm. This, too, will re-sult in a decreased cardiac output and in its severe form can result in failure of the effectiveness of the heart as a pump.

Rhythm of Death

Pacemakers in the ventricles can also set up a fibrillatory activity similar to that described for the atria. This causes the ventricles to twitch and squirm without producing any effective contraction. As a result, in the absence of any significant forceful ventricular con-traction, no blood is pumped out of the heart and cardiac output drops to zero. The blood pressure is unobtainable and life is threatened. An individual who has ventricular fibrillation can live only a few minutes unless the abnormality is corrected or other measures are taken to maintain adequate circulation to the brain and other vital areas of the body.

What Skipped Beats Mean and How to Stop Them

Simple premature contractions or extra beats may be seen in al-most any normal, healthy individual. A large number of these were documented in active flyers of the United States Air Force. These represented premature contractions originating from either the atria or the ventricles. It is a fairly safe assumption that almost everyone at one time or another has occasional irregularities of the heartbeat of this type. Despite their occurrence in normal individ-uals, they can be disabling and cause discomfort or annoyance, even though no disease is present. Often they are found to be stimulated by the excessive use of tobacco and coffee, or in individuals with high levels of nervous tension. Sometimes they are stimulated by indigestion. An individual who is having frequent episodes of extra beats would be well advised to discontinue the use of tobacco, coffee, and other stimulants—treat his digestive tract kindly and attempt to remove any other apparent causes for nervous tension that may be obvious—provided he wishes to relieve himself of the symptoms. Otherwise he must learn to live with them. Extra beats in the atria sometimes precede more significant abnormalities of the heartbeat such as atrial fibrillation. Ventricular premature contractions or extrasystoles are more common than those originating from the atria, and the general remarks concerning habits and prevention previously stated apply to them as well.

When extra beats occur for the first time, in a significant number, or in increasing numbers, they may indicate the presence of underlying heart disease. A change in their character and frequency often gives the physician a clue to the impending possibility of ventricular tachycardia or ventricular fibrillation. Under these circumstances the doctor may elect to use medications known to suppress the extra beats, thereby preventing these auxiliary pacemakers from gaining control of the heart or precipitating more serious abnormalities of the heartbeat.

Rapid Heart Palpitation May Be Curable

Atrial tachycardia may occur in normal individuals without underlying heart disease. The cause is not always detectable. Such episodes happen suddenly. The heartbeat may be regular and totally unnoticed by the person until the sudden onset of rapid heart action. The rate of the heart during such an episode will strongly influence the amount of difficulty the person will experience. If the rate is very rapid the pumping action of the heart may be compromised and the patient may feel faint. Not infrequently such episodes stop as abruptly as they begin. Some are definitely related to excessive amounts of coffee or tobacco, and occasionally to excessive ingestion of alcohol. Some individuals who have arrhythmias of this type have overactive thyroids. When this is the case, proper diagnosis and treatment can prevent recurrence. The vast majority of these disturbances in the heartbeat, however, do not appear to have any underlying cause and many of them recur at irregular or unpredictable intervals.

Preventive administration of certain medications on a regular basis is indicated when episodes of palpitation occur too frequently or are incapacitating. Most of these medications are related to, or have the same action as, quinine. These medications suppress the activity of the auxiliary pacemakers.

Individuals who are subject to rapid heart action, such as atrial tachycardia, cannot be permitted to engage in sensitive occupations. Even though no heart disease may be present, the abnormal functioning of the heart as a pump during such episodes may cause an individual to faint or otherwise be incapable of functioning properly. For this reason, individuals with such irregularities of the heart are not allowed to fly airplanes, nor should they be allowed to drive school buses, railroad locomotives, and commercial transport buses, or to engage in any other activity in which it is absolutely essential that they be conscious and able to function in a normal manner at all times. This precaution is not only to protect the individual, even though that is important, but to protect the rest of the public or school children from becoming victims of his handicap. There are many other places that individuals with these types of difficulties can function adequately and well.

Some attacks of rapid heart action, particularly those occurring from a pacemaker in the atria, can be stopped by stimulating nerves which inhibit the heart rate. Sometimes taking a deep breath and holding it will stimulate the nerves to slow the heartbeat, stopping the rapid heart action abruptly. Gagging by sticking the fingers in the back of the throat will stimulate the same reflexes and may cause the abnormal rapid heart action to cease. Physicians have used other means, such as pressing upon the eyeballs which will stimulate the same reflex mechanisms, or stimulating the artery in the neck (*carotid artery*). In some individuals simply lightly touching the neck artery in the right spot will result in a dramatic cessation of the rapid heart action with immediate relief of all discomfort and symptoms. This maneuver is not recommended for individuals who are not skilled in its application. In older individuals compression of the neck artery can cause a stroke by occluding the blood supply to the brain. This is particularly apt to occur in older people because many of them already have impaired blood flow to the brain caused by diseased arteries. Perhaps the best maneuver for use by an untrained person is to lie down in a comfortable position, take a very deep breath and hold it for as long as possible before releasing it. If this does not stop the episode, it may be tried again. Any individual who is having such episodes, however, should at the first opportunity seek medical attention for a complete examination.

The curious rhythm called atrial fibrillation, which causes the atria to beat at rates of around five hundred beats per minute may, oddly enough, occur in relatively healthy people. These are rare individuals who may live an average life span, living a completely normal life. In such instances the irregularity usually occurs as short episodes or attacks. Between attacks the heart mechanism is perfectly normal. If the ventricular contractions are slow, at a relatively normal rate, an individual can have such episodes without being aware of their occurrence. After all, the heart pumps a normal amount of blood, and if the different mechanisms to distribute it to the brain and other areas are normal, there is no reason for the atrial fibrillation to cause any disturbance in body function. If a demand is placed upon the heart to increase its cardiac output, such as during severe exertion or other moments of stress, the presence of atrial fibrillation can seriously handicap the maximum ability of the heart to function as a pump.

If too many of the rapid impulses from the atria suddenly begin to be transmitted to the ventricles, they may beat very rapidly and ineffectively. This may even result in heart failure and sudden death of the individual. The difficulty in evaluating this problem in individuals is twofold. First, making certain there is not some form of underlying heart disease; and second, determining that when atrial fibrillation occurs it will not cause a significant impairment in the heart's ability as a pump. Should the latter event occur, the individual might have fainting episodes or shock, or might die even though there is no underlying evidence of heart disease.

The vast majority of people with atrial fibrillation do have some form of disease. Some of the episodes are due to abnormal thyroid function and in other instances the attacks are associated with acute illnesses, such as pneumonia or other infections. The most common cause of atrial fibrillation is our old friend the great killer —atherosclerotic disease of the coronary arteries. Not infrequently some individuals who exhibit atrial fibrillation have had recent heart attacks.

An Astronaut's Atrial Twitch

The capriciousness of the problem of atrial fibrillation is well exemplified by some of the cases I saw in the Air Force flying population. One of these was the celebrated case of Astronaut Donald "Deke" Slayton. When he first entered the nation's astronaut program his heart rate was normal and there was no evidence that he had any form of cardiac disease or abnormal heart function.

Later he was found to have intermittent episodes of atrial fibrillation. The heart rate was usually slow when these occurred and, although he learned to detect their presence, at no time did these intermittent episodes cause him any major difficulties. He was able to exercise and carry on a normal life pattern, the same as other active individuals. He was examined while running on the treadmill at high levels of cardiac work, even in the presence of atrial fibrillation. Although his condition ruled out the possibility of his making an orbital space flight, he, like many other persons with so-called idiopathic* atrial fibrillation, has continued to lead a normal life.

The Secretive General

About the same time that Astronaut Slayton experienced his difficulties, an Air Force General in his early forties who appeared to be in good health developed persistent atrial fibrillation for the first time. Although he denied any difficulties or problems it was later learned that he had experienced an acute heart attack. Shortly after his atrial fibrillation was discovered, at a time when he would normally have been flying a large Strategic Air Command jet bomber, he dropped dead suddenly at his desk. An examination disclosed the presence of the great killer and the cause of his atrial fibrillation—namely coronary artery disease.

The Forty-Year Twitch

Atrial fibrillation may occur only once or twice in a lifetime, associated with specific circumstances. A common cause is over indulgence in alcohol. New Year's Day is a good time for the occur-

* The term *idiopathic* is a fancy medical term meaning "I don't know the cause."

rence of atrial fibrillation, and I have seen a number of cases following a New Year's Eve debauch. These usually disappear spontaneously with adequate rest and reassurance.

An example of the problem that the doctor has in evaluating the causes of atrial fibrillation was exemplified by a colonel in the Air Force whom I once saw with this problem. He was a very pleasant officer and had led an exemplary career. The time of his fortieth birthday was at hand, and like many men he viewed the approach of this anniversary with some misgiving. The evening before his birthday, he had gone to the officers' club for a party, where he consumed more than his fair share of alcohol. The following day he continued his work as usual but felt extremely tired. He had planned to return home, have a quiet dinner, and retire early. When he got home he found that his neighbors and friends had come to have a surprise birthday party to celebrate the occasion. Not wishing to be a party pooper, he promptly took a pep pill and proceeded to enjoy the festivities of the evening. Finally, the last drink was downed and the last friend had gone home. Since he was forty and didn't wish to see his masculine powers fade with the advance of age, he took his wife to bed and during the night achieved two orgasms.

The following morning, somewhat weakened by the previous night of debauch and lack of sleep, he arose, went to the bathroom, shaved, and prepared himself for his day's work. He decided to take a tub bath to try to recuperate from all that had happened. While resting in the tub, he suddenly felt his heart begin to beat irregularly and rapidly. He was weak and sweaty. He felt so bad that he went to see the doctor, who made a diagnosis of atrial fibrillation. With conservative management, the irregularity of his heartbeat disappeared.

When this case was brought to my attention, concerning the advisability of his continuing flying duties, I considered that he would probably not have another fortieth birthday, and indeed that the event could be a satisfactory one-time cause for atrial fibrillation. Not too long after I had championed his cause and had succeeded in obtaining a favorable ruling for his return to flying status, he again sustained an episode of atrial fibrillation. I thought this was really the end—surely this was sufficient cause to remove him from flying activities.

To my amazement he had still a second story. Once again his social activities had been his undoing. Friends had visited him and he had had a few extra drinks of alcohol, although he had been somewhat leery of this practice after his earlier experience. While driving from an adjacent airport toward town, his wife had suddenly developed cardiac arrest—her heart had stopped beating. While his friend drove he provided external cardiac massage to his wife on the way to the emergency room of the hospital. This requires considerable vigorous physical activity on the part of the individual administering the cardiac massage. Finally they arrived at the emergency room and it was confirmed that his wife was in cardiac arrest. She was properly treated and her life saved. In the wake of this trying experience, the colonel felt weak and asked the doctor to check him over too. He was found once again to have atrial fibrillation.

First, I checked upon the veracity of his story, which amazingly enough turned out to be true. Once again, I thought that this was a very unusual circumstance. He repeatedly denied that he had ever noticed any such episodes during severe physical exertion, so that probably the emotional stress of the occasion had precipitated his fibrillation.

As a final check, however, I decided to increase the level of his exercise done as part of our testing procedure. During the course of his increasing level of exercise, fibrillation occurred again. This left me with no other choice than to assume that he was an individual who was susceptible under different levels of stress to acute atrial fibrillation. Such an individual, regardless of the general status of his health, could not be permitted to fly jet aircraft or to engage in other sensitive occupations that required him to be in optimal health at all times.

Cheating Death

Ventricular fibrillation is a death-dealing irregularity unless it is corrected. When a person dies from being struck by lightning, ventricular fibrillation is usually the cause. The sudden heart attack, due to the great killer, often precipitates such an irregularity. The exact way in which it is triggered by a heart attack is not clearly understood, but it is directly related to a sudden inadequate blood supply to part of the heart muscle. Often the amount of muscle damage caused by a heart attack may be relatively small or nonexistent, but the occurrence of ventricular fibrillation causes sudden death.

When ventricular fibrillation occurs, if the individual is fortunate and others trained in providing cardiac massage are immediately available, his life may be saved. Sufficient circulation may be maintained as long as breathing is continued and adequate regular compression of the chest is achieved. By pressing the breastbone or sternum down against the spine, the ventricular chambers of the heart are compressed. The blood within the ventricles is pressed out of the heart into the great arteries. As pressure is released from the chest, the heart expands, permitting more blood to drain into the ventricles. Circulation may be maintained for an appreciable length of time by recurrent pumping action of this type, even though the ventricles are fibrillating in an ineffective manner. If an airway is not kept open so that the lungs are ventilated properly, the circulating blood will not be picking up oxygen and death will ensue anyway—or the patient will suffer brain damage.

The administration of external cardiac massage is a relatively simple procedure and can be carried out by individuals with a minimal amount of training. *Considering the number of individuals who die from heart attacks and ventricular fibrillation as opposed to the number of individuals who die from drowning, the most important resuscitation procedure for individuals to know today is not artificial respiration but external cardiac massage.*

By delivering an appropriate electrical shock to the ventricular muscle, the fibrillatory activity can be stopped entirely. The shock may cause momentary cardiac standstill. It is necessary to stop the fibrillation, however, before a normal beating mechanism can be restored. The heart may be stimulated electrically to resume its normal beating mechanism after the fibrillation has stopped. This can usually be accomplished, thereby restoring the normal automatic pumping action of the heart. An immediately available adequate means of controlling the heartbeat would prevent many of the deaths caused by the great killer.

You Can Stop Your Heart

Cardiac arrest is a distinct entity, separate from ventricular fibrillation. It occurs when the primary atrial pacemaker and all subsidiary pacemakers cease to fire—to stimulate the heartbeat.

When this occurs there is no evidence of electrical activity generated from the heart and no effective heartbeat. Interestingly enough, this can be induced temporarily in normal people, by breathholding or by other mechanisms used to stimulate the nerve reflex mechanisms that slow or inhibit the heart. The heart may stop during simple fainting, regardless of whether the faint is induced by prolonged upright standing, by fright, or by a needle prick. Obviously, whenever the heart stops it is no longer effective as a pump. Blood pressure falls, and unless resuscitation is accomplished death ensues.

Heart Fits

Sometimes there are abnormalities in transmitting the electrical impulse from the atria to the ventricles. These are usually caused by failure of the ventricular pacemaker's ability to transmit such an impulse. If the impulse is simply delayed, but eventually transmitted (*partial heart block*), it may not cause any significant abnormality in heart function; this can be observed even in healthy individuals. When the impulse is completely interrupted it is called *complete heart block* and is often due to some form of heart disease—commonly our old friend coronary artery disease. In this event, the atrial reservoirs and the ventricular chambers beat independently of each other—the atria beating along at their own rate, stimulated by the atrial pacemaker, while the ventricles beat along at their own rate, stimulated by a ventricular pacemaker. The pumping action of the ventricles is compromised and the amount of blood pumped by the heart may be limited when the ventricles beat very slowly. This is true particularly for those individuals who have underlying heart disease and whose ventricular muscle is not in a strong condition to begin with, because of extensive atherosclerotic disease of the coronary arteries.

Patients will lose consciousness or have convulsive seizures if ineffective heartbeats do not provide adequate blood flow to the brain. During convulsive seizures, the ventricles may actually be in arrest or having a bout of ventricular fibrillation. Specialized equipment has made it possible to record the electrical activity of the heart on a relatively continuous basis. Such recordings have demonstrated that some individuals with this problem may have transitory episodes of ventricular fibrillation, which disappear on their own. These are of very short duration and are invariably accompanied by symptoms of faintness, weakness, or near shock. If the irregularity peristed the patient would die. Mechanisms are now available for treating a large number of people who have heart block. There are implantable pacemakers which are capable of controlling the heartbeat independent of the disease of the natural pacemakers. The ability to monitor heartbeat activity on a continuous basis, the means to defibrillate electrically the fibrillating ventricles, methods of pacing the hearbeat automatically, as well as the advances of surgery, have all added a new chapter to maintaining the function of the heart as a pump. These techniques have saved or prolonged the lives of many—making new and dramatic advances in treating heart disease.

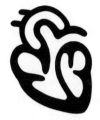

CHAPTER V

Environment Affects Circulation

MAN'S CIRCULATION is adapted to function as a transport mechanism for an "earthling." Changes in the environment, such as encountered in manned space flights, require new adaptations which influence the function of the heart and circulation.

Circulatory problems were a major consideration in bombing dives during World War II. When man left sea level to fly airplanes at increasing altitudes, he soon learned that his circulation wasn't designed for these purposes. Man must make adaptations to new environments or the environment must be controlled by an external device such as the pressurized jet aircraft, the submarine or the space capsule. The earth is a giant spaceship, spinning upon its own axis as it orbits about the sun. The external atmosphere, surrounding the giant space station, shields the surface of the earth from the harmful radiation of outer space. The gravity field surrounding the planet gives objects the characteristic of weight.

Gravity has a major influence on the blood pressure in different regions of the body if one is standing upright as opposed to lying down. This amazing environmental factor influences the amount of water in the body, the distribution of blood, and even the function of the kidneys. Failure of the circulation to adapt to gravity when an individual stands upright results in simple fainting. There is a zone of external pressure surrounding the planet earth called *atmospheric pressure*. At sea level this is equivalent to 760 mmHg, or fifteen pounds per square inch. This pressure is essential to maintain the proper amount of oxygen and other gases necessary for life as we know it. Gravity, pressure, percentage of gases, heat, cold, radiation, and many other factors constitute an environmental envelope about the surface of the earth—capable of sustaining life.

Standing up Changes Blood Pressure

Pressure at the bottom of a column of fluid depends upon the height of the column. A good example is the town water tower creating pressure for a water system by virtue of its height above the ground. Blood within the arteries and veins obeys the same principle. The pressure exerted by an upright column of blood depends upon its height and is caused by gravity. A column of blood as tall as an average man exerts a pressure of approximately 100 mmHg. Since this pressure behaves like a water column it is called *hydrostatic pressure,* and it is unrelated to the pumping action of the heart. The blood pressure while standing is a combination of both factors.

The pressure at the aortic valve—*heart-level pressure*—is independent of gravity, but is increased at all points below the aortic valve because of gravity.

Gravity decreases the blood pressure at the brain. In an adult male, the distance between the heart and the top of the skull is about twelve inches. A column of blood of this height creates a pressure of 24 mmHg. The heart must pump blood upward against this pressure, when one is seated or standing. Arterial pressure can be affected throughout the body by changing body position. While lying down, there are no tall upright columns of blood and the pressure in the different parts of the arterial tree is about the same as that at heart level.

Hydrostatic pressure affects venous and arterial pressure the same way, so that flow from the high pressure arterial system to the low pressure venous system is unchanged. The large elastic venous reservoir above the heart readily accommodates all of the venous blood that can be drained from the head and upper extremities back to the heart. The veins in the arms will collapse if you are seated upright and raise the arm above the head. In a similar fashion the veins in the neck also collapse to a point just above the level where they enter into the large right atrial reservoir.

Blood Pools in the Legs

The capacity of the venous circulation is very large and the vessels are easily distended. When you stand up, the veins in your legs expand. When you lie down and raise the legs above the head, these veins will collapse or may seem to disappear. While standing, the large veins of the leg muscles and those in the abdomen expand to accommodate more of the total blood volume. As the large veins below the heart distend with blood, less blood is available for circulation. The venous reservoir acts as a natural lake. This effect is called *venous pooling.* If the blood "pools" without a sufficient exchange of new blood, the hemoglobin in the red blood cells loses more oxygen and the blood turns dark in color. The dark unoxygenated blood may cause a bluish discoloration of the skin— *cyanosis.*

The amount of blood that can pool in the legs and thighs depends a lot on the amount of external pressure provided by the tissues around the veins. If the muscle tissue around the veins is tight and firm, the expansion of the veins is limited. Soft muscles without tone do not provide much external support to the veins to prevent their expansion. If too much blood pools in the lower part of the body, there will not be enough blood returned to the heart for normal pumping action. Then the output from the heart falls and the person may faint. Elastic bandages from the toes to above the knees, elastic stockings, or other external pressure devices prevent overexpansion of the veins and fainting.

There are numerous small valves in the veins which work like the locks on a canal. Their function is to prevent blood from flowing backward and to assist in returning blood to the heart. The valves of dilated or damaged veins may not work efficiently, causing excessive pooling of blood in the legs. These large dilated *varicose veins* are common and often require surgical correction. Pressure bandages, lying down and elevating the feet above the heart, or surgical correction, are all designed to prevent pooling of blood in the legs, causing inadequate circulation to the tissues.

Heart Function Changes with Standing

Because venous pooling occurs while standing, the amount of blood returning to the heart is decreased in normal people. This decreases the amount of blood in the individual chambers of the heart and its over-all size. There is less blood in the right and left ventricular cavities. Each heartbeat ejects less blood, or in technical terms the stroke volume is decreased. The heart responds by increasing its rate. When these mechanisms are optimally balanced, the amount of blood pumped by the heart (cardiac output) is decreased slightly. The circulation has to transport the same amount of oxygen—lying or standing. This is accomplished by each unit of circulating blood giving up more oxygen on its trip around the body. The ability to increase the removal of oxygen from the circulating blood is made possible by another of nature's redundant mechanisms.

Pumping Blood Uphill and Downhill

If there were no reflexes to change the size of the arteries, standing would cause most of the cardiac output to flow downhill into the legs and lower portions of the body and there would not be enough pressure to cause blood flow uphill to the brain. Through reflex mechanisms, a signal is sent to the small arteries, and the muscular tube around each artery contracts, decreasing the size of the opening in the arteries to the lower part of the body. This mechanism prevents the blood from all flowing directly to the legs and maintains blood flow to the brain. This reflex action is one of man's adaptations to gravity and enables him to stand upright.

While standing, the body uses its cardiac output more efficiently by changing the blood flow to different parts of the body. The amount of blood flowing to the kidney, liver, abdomen, and legs is significantly decreased. The blood flow to the heart muscle and brain is relatively unchanged.

Airplanes and Space Launching

Anyone who has ridden in an elevator or a roller coaster has experienced the sensation of changes in acceleration. When the elevator zooms upward the natural inertia of the blood causes it to move footward. As a roller coaster starts back up the incline, pulling out of the dip gives one's body a sense of increased weight, pushing it down into the seat. This causes the blood to weigh more and increases the blood pressure in the lower part of the body while decreasing it at levels above the heart.

By the time the United States entered into World War II, new aircraft had been developed for high-speed bombing missions. The airplane screamed downward toward its target and, at the bottom of this dive, dropped its bombs and then pulled up sharply. The U-turn, caused by the diving maneuver, is an exaggeration of the roller coaster effect. If the pull-up of the airplane was too sharp, the wings would snap off the airplane. The wings of the planes, however, were much stronger than man's ability to withstand these effects. When the force created by pulling out of the bombing dive was too great, the reflex controls for the distribution of the circulation could no longer cope with the problem and most of the blood would go to the lower portion of the body with inadequate amounts of blood or none being pumped to the brain. With luck the pilot merely lost his vision temporarily. Greater forces caused the pilot to black out.

Soon man learned how to improve his circulatory tolerance to these events. By leaning forward from the hips, so that the long axis of the trunk was parallel with the long axis of the plane, the pilot could pull out of steeper dives. Leaning forward decreased the height of the column of blood from the top of the head to the hips, diminishing the dive's effect.

The peculiarities of the circulation require astronauts to be launched into space lying down. The rocket force required to accelerate a spacecraft upward and outward at sufficient speed to orbit about the earth is much larger than the forces that had previously been encountered in aircraft. If the astronauts were seated upright, this force would increase the weight of the column of blood in the body to such a degree that there would certainly be no circulation to the brain. The obvious solution was to have the astronauts lie down on their backs, thereby making the long tubular aorta parallel with the surface of the earth—essentially eliminating any tall columns of blood. This minimized the pressure changes created by the weight of the blood during the rocket thrust required to obtain orbital velocity.

Once the astronaut is in orbit, there is no effective gravity force on the space capsule. The arterial and venous pressures then are related simply to the pumping action of the heart and to variations in the size of the arteries and veins. The effects of "weight-lessness" on circulation are very similar to the effects of bed rest. Despite the tremendous speed of the space vehicle, the astronaut is able to sit up or change body position without any significant alteration of the circulation. In the absence of a significant gravitational force, or weight, body position is no longer of any consequence as far as the circulation is concerned.

During re-entry, the space vehicle is again positioned so that the forces created by the rapid slowdown of the space vehicle are perpendicular to the long axis of the body and well within man's tolerance. The story of aerial and space flight exemplifies the importance of body position in relationship to the function of the heart and circulation.

Gaining Weight While Standing Around

The increase in arterial and venous pressure while standing increases the migration of fluid out of the vascular tree into the tissue spaces. The extra fluid is stored in spaces underneath the skin, between and in the muscles. Measurements taken of the circumference of the thigh and leg in healthy individuals during quiet standing have demonstrated the gradual increase in their size. Muscles are bound in membranous sheaths, much like a canvas water bag. When this sheath is tough and tight about the muscle, it will limit the extent of expansion. This, in turn, will limit the amount of water which can be literally poured into the muscle sac. In muscles with tight outer linings, the internal pressure increases. The increased firmness of water-filled muscles exerts increased external pressure around the great veins in the legs, helping to prevent venous pooling. Where the tissue is loose or there is not such a tight covering, the muscles and tissues continue to fill with additional water.

In order to maintain blood volume, additional water must be stored in the body. If the water level is low, one drinks more water and the kidneys excrete less water until an adequate balance is achieved. Increased loading of the body with water is one of the adaptations we make to the upright position. Hence, the normal person who is walking around in his daily activities weighs about five pounds more than the person who has been in bed for a few days. This is one of the factors that causes the body weight to be normally higher at the end of the day than it is in the morning when you first get up.

Losing Weight While Resting in Bed

It took the space age to stimulate a second look at the influence of bed rest and its effects upon the circulation. For generations, physicians have been putting people to bed as part of the treatment for everything from colds to heart attacks. Yet, only a handful of studies had ever been done on the effects of bed rest on apparently healthy people—six men had been studied at the University of Minnesota and four at Cornell University. Almost all other studies were done in patients with illnesses or injuries that precluded the possibility of learning how bed rest affected man. Bed rest was studied in a large number of normal subjects because the effects were very similar to those expected in manned space flights. The results of these studies showed that bed rest is not necessarily a good thing. The human body was not made to lie around in bed. Bed rest results in the deterioration of the body whether or not disease is present.

When a normally active person goes to bed the blood which was pooled below the diaphragm shifts into the thorax. The amount of blood in the lungs and thoracic area is significantly increased. The great right and left atrial reservoirs expand to accommodate the increased volume of blood returning to the heart. There is a set of complex detectors imbedded in the wall of the atria that sense the stretching of the atrial wall caused by the increased volume. These are called *stretch receptors*. Through a reflex mechanism, they send a signal to the brain, relaying the information that the left atrium has more blood in it than it needs. In turn, the brain relays the signal to the pituitary gland, just underneath it. This complex little gland has many functions, including secreting hormones that control human growth and the functions of the other endocrine glands. One of its functions is to regulate the amount of water excreted by the kidney. A hormone secreted by the pituitary limits the amount of water the kidney filters out of the bloodstream. The signal from the brain, when a person is lying down, literally stops the pituitary gland from secreting this hormone.

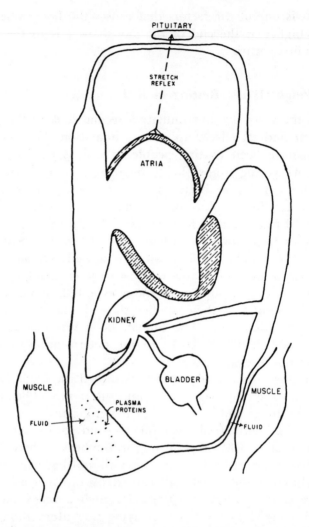

This, in turn, frees the kidneys to speed up their rate of eliminating water from the body. This process gradually decreases the blood volume as well as the amount of blood in the large atrial reservoirs that stimulated the stretch receptors.

Upon lying down, the increased hydrostatic pressure that caused storage of water in the muscles and tissues in the lower part of the body, is no longer present. Water from the tissues outside of the vascular tree returns to the circulation and maintains the blood volume. As long as this continues, the stretch receptors in the atrial reservoirs are stimulated and the body continues to pour out water from the kidneys. When the process is complete, the water in the plasma is also reduced, thereby decreasing the total blood volume. As far as the water and salt content of the body is concerned, the body is then adapted to bed rest. Usually the amount of excess water which is poured out during simple recumbency by a normally active individual will weigh approximately five pounds and will be reflected in an appropriate loss of body weight.

The loss of water from the plasma causes the circulating blood to become more concentrated. Initially, the number of red blood cells is unchanged and the loss of water results in an increased number of red blood cells per unit of blood volume. This can easily be detected by simple laboratory measurements on the number of red blood cells in the blood. *The initial loss of weight from simple bed rest has nothing to do with calories or loss of fat tissue. It is a partial dehydration or loss of water from the body which is quickly replaced once normal activity is resumed.*

Astronauts Lose Weight in Space

The Mercury and Gemini astronauts lost weight during orbital flights. In some instances, this was related to increased heat loads and other environmental factors, but when these conditions were controlled, weight loss was still observed. This was anticipated from the studies of young healthy people at bed rest. Upon returning to earth, with normal ambulatory activities, all of the astronauts quickly regained their weight, much of which was achieved by replenishing water lost from the body tissues.

Getting Out of Bed May Be a Problem

Ordinarily you cannot blame recumbency during a simple night's sleep for your reluctance to get out of bed in the morning, but if you are in bed for two days or longer, you may be in for some surprises when you get up. An interval of forty-eight hours is long enough for the loss of body water from bed rest to occur. After that, the water balance levels off with the intake and output of water essentially in balance. The reflexes that normally cause the arteries in the lower part of the body to contract on standing are not stimulated during bed rest and may grow sluggish. A basic principle of life is, *if you don't use it, you lose it.*

The loss of water diminishes the amount of circulating blood volume available for a transport mechanism. Because of the loss of water stored in the muscles and tissues in the lower part of the body, the muscles lose tone and become weak and flabby, failing to exert any significant pressure on the large venous reservoir. Upon standing upright, the reflex mechanism to constrict the arteries in the lower part of the body may not work well enough, causing difficulty in maintaining enough pressure to send blood to the brain. The loss of muscle tone and body water allows the large venous reservoir to expand unduly so it can accommodate a greater amount of blood volume than before. Since there is less blood volume anyway, the increased venous pooling may seriously limit the amount of blood which can be returned to the heart for circulation. The absence of the normal amount of water stores in the muscles and tissues causes an increased outpouring of water from the circulation into these tissues. These combined effects result in greatly compromising the circulation's ability to provide blood to the brain. Hence, many individuals after periods of bed rest feel faint and weak when they first get up. If proper precautions are not taken, some can and do faint. Faintness of this type was observed in a number of the astronauts on their return to earth after orbital space flight.

The practicing physician has long been aware of the tendency to faintness after prolonged periods of bed rest. Sometimes this is erroneously attributed to the illness, when actually the bed rest alone is the culprit. The proper amount of water can be restored to the tissues, the blood volume increased, and the various reflex mechanisms reactivated in a gradual manner. Usually the patient is asked to sit up on the edge of the bed for fifteen minutes the first day and dangle his feet. The next day there may be two or three intervals, then gradually the length and frequency of the intervals are increased. Finally, the patient sits up in a chair and ultimately resumes his normal walking habits. With this gradual exposure to the normal stresses of the effects of earth's gravitational force, a person is gradually readapted to normal upright activity.

The simple act of walking goes a long way in preventing fainting from bed rest or other causes, when venous pooling is a major factor.

The contraction of the leg muscles literally squeezes the venous reservoir and milks blood back to the heart. Motionless standing without contracting the muscles contributes to fainting, but walking or contracting the muscles acts as an auxiliary pump and is a protective mechanism.

Bed Rest May Weaken Your Heart

When there is a real need for it, bed rest is a very important part of medical treatment. This is particularly true when the circulatory system is not functioning properly and shock results. There are times when it is important to rest the heart, although this can be done seated upright nearly as well as lying down. The late Dr. Samuel Levine championed the chair treatment of acute heart attacks as opposed to the old-fashioned treatment of absolute bed rest for six weeks. The pressure created by the column of blood from the heart to the top of the head helps to fill the coronary arteries and no doubt this increased pressure helps to maintain blood flow to the injured heart muscle after a heart attack. Of course, chair rest is not used if the patient has shock or other problems which dictate that he should be in bed.

One of the ways to test the efficiency of the circulation is to have a person exercise to his maximum capability. The increased work involved requires that more oxygen be transported by the circulation. In endurance exercises, like running, the factor limiting exercise capacity for moderately active healthy people is usually the heart's ability to pump blood to the lungs. For this reason, measuring the maximum amount of oxygen that can be absorbed by the body, or transported by the blood, is an index of the effectiveness of the circulation. Numerous exercise studies of young men after prolonged bed rest, carried out by the United States Air Force, demonstrated that bed rest decreased the capacity of the circulation to transport blood and decreased the amount of work that a normal person could do. Prolonged bed rest often results in a gradual and progressive increase of the heart rate, even while the individual is still in bed. As discussed earlier, increasing the heart rate decreases the efficiency of the heart muscle. Each contraction requires that the heart overcome the inertia of the muscle fibers. As the heart rate increases, the heart tends to decrease in size. The longer the period of bed rest and its associated inactivity, the more likely the heart is to become small with a rapid rate. The small rapidly beating heart is an inefficient heart, frequently not capable of meeting the stresses of normal active life.

One should not overemphasize the adverse effects of bed rest. In the past, patients with tuberculosis frequently spent months and sometimes years at prolonged bed rest. Despite this, their greatest problem was tuberculosis and not bed rest. Under normal circumstances, the major difficulties associated with bed rest occur when the person gets out of bed and these difficulties can be controlled.

There are other complications which may occur during bed rest, including the formation of blood clots in the veins of the legs and lower body which may be released and carried to the lungs or vital organs. Such episodes usually cause a medical emergency and may result in nearly instantaneous death.

In general, unless the illness is of a nature to require bed rest, the patient is much better off sitting in a chair or restricting his activity. Respiratory infections and a host of minor illnesses are not an adequate reason for bed rest. Coddling one's self in bed through several days of minor illness, merely adds to the general weakness, fatigue, and debilitation that follows in the wake of such an illness, and much of this weakness is directly related to the change in function of the circulatory system.

That "Old Blood" Feeling

Many individuals experience fatigue for days after unusual activity. This also occurs on resuming activity after bed rest. Young healthy men frequently developed a mild anemia upon returning to normal activity. Red blood cells can be destroyed by mechanical action. The more they are vibrated, shaken, or blasted against the vessel walls, the more likely they are to be destroyed. Each day a certain number of cells are destroyed by the normal activity of living. These are replenished by the blood-forming organs such as the bone marrow. A balance develops between the blood cells produced and those destroyed. As long as this balance is evenly maintained, there is not likely to be an anemia.

During bed rest, the normal mechanical actions which destroy the red blood cells are grossly limited, and many of them live longer. The stimulus for the blood-forming organs to create new red blood cells is markedly diminished. Once a person gets out of bed and begins to exercise, the usual causes for destruction of red blood cells resume. The old blood cells are rapidly and precipitously destroyed. The blood-forming organs which have been idle cannot provide sudden massive replacements, since the bone marrow gradually regains its ability to replace red blood cells. While the cells are being destroyed, and the bone marrow is not up to optimal production, there is a sharp drop in the amount of red blood cells in the circulating blood. This type of anemia is usually corrected within two or three weeks in healthy people.

Altitude Can Make Your Heart Work Harder

The effects of altitude upon the circulation are recorded in ancient writings. These early descriptions have been erroneously confused with chest pain originating from the heart, later known as angina pectoris. A description of exposure to altitude in the Alps by Coelius Aurelianus, as quoted by William Heberden, is classical for the effects of decreased oxygen associated with altitude. The following is an excerpt from this description. "A peculiar tiredness often comes upon those who are ascending such high hills, so that it is impossible to proceed four steps further; and if it were attempted, such strong universal palpitations would come on, as could not fail to end in swooning."

As one progresses to higher and higher altitudes, the atmospheric pressure gradually decreases below that found at sea level. The thinner air contains less oxygen. At sea level the oxygen in the atmosphere creates a pressure of 159.60 mmHg (760 mmHg x 21% =159.60 mmHg). The percentage of oxygen in the atmosphere remains unchanged, but the atmosphere's pressure decreases with increasing altitude. This has the same effect as if one were breathing air with a lower percentage of oxygen at sea level. An idea of the effect may be obtained by considering the effects of altitude at different geographical locations. Breathing air at Denver, Colorado, with an altitude of five thousand feet, is similar to breathing an air mixture with only eighteen per cent oxygen at sea level, compared to the normal twenty-one per cent. If you go to Mexico City, with an altitude of approximately seven thousand feet, breathing air will be similar to breathing a sixteen per cent oxygen mixture at sea level. At an altitude of ten thousand feet such as may be found at Leadville, Colorado, the atmospheric pressure is further decreased and the amount of oxygen is similar to a sea-level mixture containing fourteen per cent oxygen. Altitude studies have been carried out in the little mining village of Morococha, Peru, which has an altitude of over fourteen thousand feet. Here, the thin air is equivalent to a twelve per cent oxygen mixture. At eighteen thousand feet the amount of oxygen in the air is less than half of that found at sea level, or equivalent to an air mixture containing ten per cent oxygen.

As altitude increases, the amount of pressure created by oxygen decreases. This, in turn, decreases the oxygen in each air sac within the lungs. Since the pressure of oxygen dissolved in the circulating blood leaving the lungs is the same as the pressure of oxygen in the air sacs, *the amount of oxygen dissolved in the circulating plasma decreases with altitude exposure.* The ratio of oxygen combined with hemoglobin is dependent upon the pressure of oxygen dissolved in the plasma. The fall in oxygen tension results in less oxygen being carried by the hemoglobin or an over-all decrease in the oxygen content of the circulating blood. *Each unit of circulating blood at altitude carries less oxygen than at sea level.*

In normal resting individuals with good heart function, a change from sea level to ten thousand feet does not require the heart to pump very much more blood, even though there is less oxygen in the blood returned from the lungs. Nature again uses one of its redundant mechanisms. The amount of oxygen delivered by each unit of circulating bood is maintained, and the amount of oxygen in the venous blood returning from the tissues is decreased. This is made possible by the reserve oxygen that is normally carried in the venous blood.

The coronary blood flow to the heart muscle is an exception to nature's redundant mechanism. As was discussed in Chapter III, the heart muscle is the only place where nearly all of the oxygen which can be removed from the circulating blood is removed at rest. There are no residual oxygen stores to provide more oxygen for the heart muscle. When altitude exposure causes a decreased oxygen content, the blood flow to the heart muscle has to increase to maintain oxygen delivery to the heart muscle. The coronary arteries must enlarge or dilate. In normal people, exposure to altitude dilates the coronary arteries and increases blood flow to the heart muscle. The increase in blood flow required to deliver the same amount of oxygen to the heart muscle at different altitudes is as follows:

Feet	Per cent
5,000	not significant
7,000	10
10,000	15
14,000	25
18,000	40

At altitudes of fourteen thousand to eighteen thousand feet, the decreased amount of oxygen in each unit of blood is sufficient to cause the heart to increase its work. This increases the need for blood flow to the heart muscle even more. In order to maintain an appropriate delivery of oxygen, more blood must be pumped by the heart. There is an increase in heart rate and systolic pressure which indicates an increased stroke volume with each heartbeat. These changes signal the increased cardiac output used to maintain adequate delivery of oxygen to the body tissues.

Of course, if work or physical effort is required, this will have an additive affect upon the work that the heart and circulation must do under conditions of higher altitude or decreased oxygen. These factors are important in endurance athletics such as football, basketball, and long distance running events. *They are very important when the sea level heart patient considers hunting or fishing at higher altitudes.* This is one way to overextend the capacity of the heart. The best-known public example of the combined influence of altitude and exertion was President Eisenhower's first heart attack after he left his Washington office to golf, fish, and hike in the mountains of Colorado. The dangers of the combined effects of altitude and physical activity will be discussed further in conjunction with exercise. There are ways that these difficulties can be avoided or minimized. Disease of the coronary arteries may prevent dilation and limit the ability to increase blood flow to the heart muscle at a high altitude. Prolonged exercise at significantly high altitudes for these people can cause chest pain or even result in an acute heart attack.

Individuals who live at high altitudes develop adaptations to the decreased amount of oxygen. The number of red blood cells is increased. Within the limits acceptable for life, the greater the altitude the more red blood cells are produced. If the altitude is high enough there may be a greater volume of red blood cells than plasma in the circulating blood. The circulating blood gradually returns to its normal sea level characteristics if the individual leaves the high altitude for an extended period.

Altitude Can Stimulate Your Coronary Arteries

Decreased oxygen results in a greater blood flow to the normal heart muscle. The number of communications between the branches of the coronary arteries and the size of the major and smaller arteries is increased. Autopsies of patients who have had inadequate oxygen in the lungs, because of lung disease, have demonstrated the increased number of connections between the different branches of the coronary arteries. This, in effect, increases the capacity to carry blood to the heart muscle. The increased number of connections augments nature's redundant system of multiple ways to supply the heart muscle with blood. This may have a protective effect against damaging the heart muscle from coronary artery disease or a heart attack, once the increased connections are developed.

You Might Be Better Off Flying

Many people with heart disease are afraid to travel by air. Usually, this is an unrealistic fear. Even though a jet airliner may be cruising at forty to fifty thousand feet above the earth, the pressurized cabin provides protection from most of the ill-effects of altitude and decreased oxygen. The pressurized cabin, in commercial aircraft, usually maintains an altitude below seven thousand feet. The additional work required of the heart or the increased coronary blood flow during rest needed at this altitude is equivalent to the most minimal amount of exercise. This is not sufficient to cause any serious difficulty in most individuals with heart disease who are still able to walk to the corner drugstore. Fear, apprehension, excitement, and the emotion of meeting friends or relatives are greater hazards to the heart patient traveling by air than the effects of the altitude.

If a person has chronic lung disease, this may be another matter, since such individuals are already suffering from many of the same effects produced by high altitude and the aerial flight constitutes in effect an additional increase in altitude exposure. Most often the greatest hazard in air flights is not altitude, but the rich food which is served in abundant quantities that adds to the girth of your waistline and the fat deposits in the walls of your arteries. If you are interested in restricting your calories or staying on a low-fat diet, you will be wise to take your own food. Other hazards associated with air travel for heart patients are those related to handling of luggage and the pressure associated with unexpected delays or making connections. Many of these can be minimized, but in the case of most heart patients more attention should be given to these airport problems than to the actual flight itself.

A curious phenomenon is the individual who is greatly concerned about altitude in air travel but doesn't give a second thought to driving his automobile across the mountains or taking a bus trip over mountainous peaks. Some highways reach altitudes of ten thousand feet or more, creating a significantly greater stress on the heart and circulation than that of air travel. If you are traveling by automobile or bus from sea level, across mountainous territory, you would be well advised to check the altitude of the mountainous route. Additional exertion in terms of handling luggage or other activities should be scrupulously avoided by older people and cardiac patients under these circumstances, unless they are already acclimatized to high altitudes and accustomed to this type of activity.

Cold, Heat, and Humidity

The heart and circulation are directly involved in maintaining the proper temperature factors of the body. If one is exposed to cold temperatures, one way of combating the problem is to increase metabolism, thereby generating body heat. Exercise is a good way of doing this. The stepped-up metabolism requires an increased transport of oxygen by the heart and circulation. In this way cold often increases the work of the heart. Exposure to cold can also cause abnormal reflex actions and other undesirable changes in the function of the heart and circulation. It has been known to precipitate chest pain in individuals with heart disease. In general, cardiac patients should avoid excessive exposure to cold. Walking in the face of a cold wind, particularly if the coat is left open, may precipitate heart pain.

The body temperature and environment must be maintained in a very narrow range for normal function. One of the functions of the skin is to help in cooling the body when an individual is exposed to excessive heat. The circulation to the skin is increased and plays a part in the normal sweating mechanism. Heat and humidity, which interfere with dissipation of body heat, significantly increase the work of the heart. In individuals with marginal heart function, heat and humidity can be major factors in determining recovery. The simple oxygen tent often used during acute heart attacks, provides a means of controlling the temperature and the humidity. In essence, it is an envelope of air conditioning. In hot, humid climates, such an envelope can significantly decrease the load placed on the heart and improve the chances for recovery. The lesson in this for heart patients, or those who are susceptible to cardiac difficulties, is clear. If you live in a hot, humid climate, good air conditioning can be very handy if you wake up some night with a-heart attack, or in decreasing the load on the circulation if you are fortunate enough to return home from the hospital.

Food, Fat, and Fate

"It's CHOLESTEROL—all you need to do is avoid eggs." "Cutting out cholesterol isn't enough, you really have to be on a low-fat diet, and I mean low." "Body weight doesn't have any relationship to heart attacks." "My doctor says if you don't lose weight you will increase your chances of having one." "I understand that you can eat fats as long as they are those unsaturated kind—you know, the oils and the like. It isn't your blood cholesterol anyway that causes trouble. It's that other kind of fat called 'triglycerides' that's really important." "The best way to lose weight is to cut out all fats." "You can eat all you want as long as you don't eat any carbohydrates. All you need to do is eat meat and fats, you can even drink alcohol—just don't eat carbohydrates. Some people call it the drinking man's diet—works wonders!" "I've been using the grapefruit diet." "My doctor says you shouldn't eat eggs." "I understand all that you have to do is exercise." "It's really the sugar that's important."

It's no wonder if you are confused after all of those conflicting remarks. Yet, each one of these approaches has been advocated as a way to control body weight and prevent heart disease. Doctors, too, have changed their minds as new knowledge has been acquired about the influence of different diets on health. Some are simply diet fads which may appear to have results but the effect is strictly temporary. In some instances the diets that have been recommended may be really harmful to your health, to the extent of increasing the likelihood of having atherosclerotic disease.

There is more agreement at the present time on the proper diet than ever before. Although there are other factors which affect the development of atherosclerosis, probably the single most important factor is what you eat. In addition to preventing atherosclerosis, a good understanding of the effects caused by different diets is the first step in satisfactory weight control. Weight control is important in individuals with most types of heart disease. Sufficient studies have been underway long enough to demonstrate that proper dietary management significantly reduces the incidence of heart attacks. Of course a person with diabetes or liver disease, and other patients under a doctor's care, will need special handling and advice; but the vast majority of the general public can profit by knowing how to adjust their diet to control calorie intake and favorably affect fat metabolism.

The Carbohydrates

The carbohydrate group represents the chief ingredient of the diet for most of the people in the world who have a low incidence of atherosclerosis. The Okinawans, for example, eat chiefly carbohydrates found in vegetables and fruit. As with other foods, carbohydrates consist of a long chain of carbon atoms combined with hydrogen and oxygen. Carbohydrates constitute the major ingredient of most fruits, vegetables, and cereals. Ordinary sugar is a simple carbohydrate in a concentrated form. More complex carbohydrates, such as those found in vegetables, contain much "roughage." Starchy foods are carbohydrates that require further action upon them by the body before they can be used by the cells for food. Digestion of *one gram of carbohydrate will create four calories.* A lesser amount of the carbohydrate found in bulky foods is actually absorbed and used for metabolism. A spoonful of pure sugar may be completely absorbed and utilized by the body. Carbohydrate is burned in the metabolic fires more economically than any other food in terms of requiring oxygen. For this reason, using carbohydrates for fuel requires the circulation to deliver less oxygen per calorie than either proteins, fats, or alcohol. This explains why foods rich in carbohydrates are often given to individuals during prolonged endurance activity.

After carbohydrates are absorbed they may be converted to the proper form to be burned for energy. Nitrogen may be added to the carbon chain to form amino acids which are used as building blocks for protein. Carbohydrates can also be converted to fat. *It is important to appreciate that ordinary carbohydrates can be converted to either proteins or fat by the body.* Carbohydrate metabolism is chiefly regulated by the liver. The liver is responsible for converting carbohydrates to protein or fat or into a form that can be stored in the muscles (*glycogen*). The liver is able to control the level of blood glucose by calling upon its own stores of carbohydrates. The role of the liver as the regulator for the amount of circulating blood sugar is significantly affected by other factors, such as insulin and the activity of other hormones.

Proteins

The long carbon chain of proteins contains nitrogen and is broken into the amino acids. These are the building products for muscle and other body tissues. Cell growth requires protein. Meat, fish, fowl, milk, and eggs are all rich sources of protein. Metabolism of *one gram of protein, like carbohydrate, will generate four calories.* The proteins can be completely used for fuel purposes or their carbon chain can be converted to, and stored as, a fat. It is commonly stated that the diet should contain at least seventy grams (two and a half ounces) of protein per day, although many healthy people eat far less, suggesting this minimal requirement may be too high. A 325 gram (eleven and a half ounces) portion of raw lean round steak contains only seventy grams of protein. Beans are a good vegetable source for proteins.

Fats

Dietary fats have received the most attention in relationship to atherosclerosis and weight control. It is important to emphasize that *each gram of fat contains nine calories.* For this reason, a small amount of fat can produce a large number of calories.

Many technical terms in relationship to fat metabolism and food fats are not difficult to understand and are sufficiently important that you should know them. Most fats used for food exist as a fatty acid—the term "acid" referring to its chemical structure. These are often combined with another substance, which organic chemists would class as an alcohol—namely, glycerol. The glycerol and the fatty acids join together as a molecule, just as sodium and chloride join to form a molecule of salt. When there are three fatty acids combined with the glycerol it is called a *triglyceride*. The size of the individual fatty acid components depends upon the length of their carbon chain; thus, you can have fats composed of very large molecules or of smaller molecules. Some of the fatty acids are not combined with glycerols and exist in the free state. These are called *free fatty acids* and are transported in the bloodstream with albumen—one of the main blood proteins.

Cholesterol, which is included in the fat group, draws more popular attention in relationship to atherosclerosis than any other substance in food. It is really not a fat. Its large molecular size enables it to have some physical properties of a fat but chemically it is closely related to the steroids secreted by the adrenal glands, the sex glands, and other endocrine glands. *Cholesterol is manufactured by the liver from other food products.* Although a small amount of it exists in the free state in the bloodstream, most of it is combined with a protein and a small amount of triglyceride fat. The combined unit of triglyceride, cholesterol, and protein is called a *lipoprotein*. In general, the lipoproteins are divided into two subgroups, depending upon their particle size. A larger particle, called *beta-lipoprotein*, contains the largest amount of cholesterol in the bloodstream, usually about seventy-five per cent. This is the lipoprotein that has been implicated in causing atherosclerosis. The fact that it contains so much cholesterol and triglyceride is the principal reason a blood cholesterol determination is of value. The blood cholesterol level suggests the amount of beta-lipoproteins circulating in the bloodstream. The smaller lipoprotein, called *alpha-lipoprotein*, contains a much smaller amount of cholesterol and triglyceride. The alpha-lipoproteins are not thought to be as important in causing atherosclerosis.

Phospholipids are still another group of fatty substances. As the name implies, these are fat molecules that contain phosphorus. They are thought to be of particular importance by some authorities because they improve the solubility of the fat particles, or prevent the fat particles from settling out as sediment. By increasing the solubility of cholesterol and lipids they may prevent them from precipitating as particles against the arterial wall and in this way protect against the development of atherosclerosis. The ratio between cholesterol and phospholipids is sometimes used as an index to the stability or solubility of the fat products in the bloodstream. The large amount of cholesterol in the beta-lipoprotein, compared to the small amount of phospholipid, is thought to be an unfavorable ratio permitting the cholesterol component to precipitate out. The smaller amount of cholesterol in the alpha-lipoprotein provides a more favorable phospholipid ratio, causing the cholesterol within the lipoprotein to be more stable.

A concept that has received major attention in recent years is the difference between saturated and unsaturated fats. This concept is a major facet in building a correct diet. The terms, which are derived from the molecular structure of the fat chain, can easily be appreciated by considering that each carbon atom has four hands. The carbon chain is formed by each carbon atom holding hands with another—like a human chain. This leaves two hands free. If each one of these two hands holds on to a hydrogen atom, the molecular structure will be a long string of carbon atoms, joined side by side, with each carbon atom holding two hydrogen atoms. The amount of hydrogen on the chain determines whether it is a saturated or unsaturated fat. Some fat molecules do not hold a hydrogen atom with each spare hand. Instead, two carbon atoms may form a double handclasp. This double bond between the carbon atoms leaves no extra hands to hold a hydrogen atom. In such a manner the chain of carbon atoms is not filled with as many hydrogen atoms as is possible. *The fewer hydrogen atoms that are present, the more unsaturated a fat is said to be. If the entire chain is full of hydrogen atoms it is said to be saturated.*

Knowledge of the principle of adding hydrogen atoms to the carbon chain to produce a saturated fat is an important one you can use when you visit the grocery store. Many unsaturated fats have been converted to saturated ones by the process called *hydrogenation.* For example, a jar of peanut butter will say on the label "partially hydrogenated." This means that nature's naturally occuring unsaturated fat has been converted to a saturated fat by adding hydrogen atoms.

Alcohol

No discussion of food substances would be complete without mentioning alcohol. All alcoholic beverages, aside from whatever other effect they may have, contain calories. In fact, alcohol is one of the richest food stuffs. *Each gram of alcohol contains seven calories,* or nearly twice the caloric content of either carbohydrates or proteins. From a caloric point of view alone, any effort to restrict calories must include consideration of any calories ingested in the form of alcohol.

The Fat Route

In order for any form of ingested food to have an effect upon the body it first must be absorbed from the stomach and intestines. Some foods are not well absorbed and are considered as diet bulk— an example is lettuce. Before the food can be absorbed it is acted upon by the digestive juices, plus the actions of numerous bacterial organisms. Bile secreted from the liver and pancreatic juices secreted by the pancreas into the small intestine are of great importance in preparing ingested fat for absorbtion. In the absence of the digestive ferments caused by certain abnormalities of the pancreas, the fat will not be converted into a form that can be absorbed from the intestine, and it will be excreted. The bowel movements of individuals with such abnormalities are described as large and foamy, containing large quantities of fat. Many essential foodstuffs normally are dissolved in conjunction with fat and transported across the intestinal wall. These include a large number of the fat-soluble vitamins essential for good health.

The action of the intestinal wall is of the greatest importance in the transport of fat. When products pass through the intestinal wall they are picked up primarily by the lymphatic system. At this point in the process almost all of the fat is triglyceride. These large fat molecules have not yet reached the bloodstream and the milky colored lymph is carried through numerous tiny channels until it reaches one common mainstream—the lymph duct, which empties into the vena cava returning blood to the large right atrial chamber.

Immediately after a fatty meal, a large amount of these milky particles are dumped into the bloodstream from the lymph duct.

These large particles are called *chylomicrons*. They apparently have no role in the development of atherosclerosis. Chylomicrons are transported by the bloodstream to the liver. Here, once again, the liver acts as a regulating organ. Some of the triglycerides are joined with protein, cholesterol, and phospholipids to form the beta-lipoproteins, others emerge from the liver in alpha-lipoproteins. A small amount of fat emerges as free fatty acid, joined with albumen in the circulating bloodstream. The level of beta-lipoproteins and consequently the level of cholesterol is kept relatively constant by the

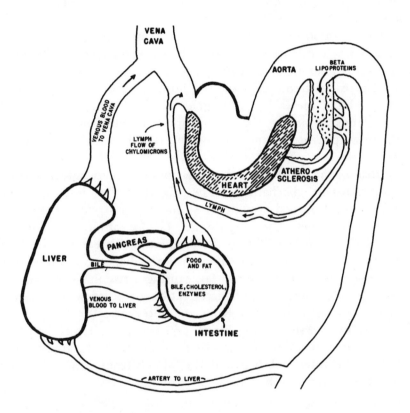

liver, just as the level of blood sugar is maintained within a narrow range. The liver is able to manufacture cholesterol. With the abilities to convert carbohydrate to fats and to manufacture cholesterol, it is clear that the liver is able to dump beta-lipoproteins into the bloodstream even in the absence of large amounts of fat in the diet. When there is not very much cholesterol in the diet, the liver often manufactures enough to maintain a fairly high blood level, even if the diet contains mostly carbohydrates and protein.

The circulating lipoproteins migrate across the blood vessel walls. Here they are again picked up by the lymph stream and transported back through the vena cava to the right atrium. If the lipoproteins accumulate in the vessel wall they produce atherosclerosis.

The control of the major mechanism for fat transport is influenced by many other body functions. Various hormones influence the mechanism. Female hormones contribute to the formation of a larger amount of alpha-lipoproteins and a lesser amount of beta-lipoproteins. The smaller amount of beta-lipoproteins is thought to be the reason the childbearing-age female is more protected from atherosclerosis than the male. The thyroid hormone tends to decrease the amount of beta-lipoprotein and the amount of cholesterol. Decreased amounts of thyroid hormone allow an elevation of these products, increasing atherosclerosis. Hormones from the adrenal glands stimulate the fat-transport mechanism to generate more beta-lipoproteins and cholesterol, thereby accelerating atherosclerosis.

Control of the function of the intestines exerts an influence upon the fat-transport mechanism. The highly active intestine with rapid transport of food provides less time for absorption. Absence of important enzymes that prepare the fat for absorption also decreases the transport of fat to the circulation. Disease of the liver can cause abnormalities in fat transport; diabetes in some way affects the ability to metabolize fat, causing a rise in the content of fat in the bloodstream, with acceleration of atherosclerosis. Hormones, diabetes, absorption from the intestines, function of the pancreas, liver disease, and blood pressure are all factors which affect the amount of atherosclerosis resulting from the transport of fat from the intestinal tract, to the bloodstream, and ultimately through the arterial wall.

The Have-Not Diet

No single dietary factor can be identified as the sole difference between the diet of the have-not people with a low incidence of atherosclerosis and that of the populations in the western industrialized nations with their very high incidence of atherosclerosis. The diet of the have-not people is different from the diet of the atherosclerotic population in many respects. The have-not diet is low in calories; in particular, the caloric intake is not in excess of the calories required for the daily energy expenditure. Under these circumstances, the body does not store calories and weight control is not a problem. The have-not diet is low in fat content. The diet of most of the have-not people is heavily based on fruits, vegetables, and cereals, and variable amounts of fish, poultry, and wild birds. For this reason, a large portion of the fat in their diet is of the unsaturated type—the vegetable oils and fish oils. The carbohydrate intake does not include the refined sugars of western civilization. Their carbohydrates consist of the starches and vegetable carbohydrates. The have-not diet is reasonably low in protein, and most of the protein source again is either vegetable, fish, or fowl in origin. Their diet also provides a very low cholesterol intake. Many of these people do have access to a ready source of fresh fruits and vegetables, permitting their diet to be rich in such vitamins as *ascorbic acid,* or vitamin C. Almost all of the have-not people are located in parts of the world where the climate is favorable for obtaining vegetables and fruit on a year-round basis. This is not true of the atherosclerotic nations where the colder winters preclude a twelve-month growing season.

Similar observations can be made about the examples of the diet in individuals with a low incidence of atherosclerosis during World War II. The well-nourished atherosclerotic people of the world were placed on diets, similar to those of the have-not nations—low in calories, low in fats, low in refined sugars, but heavy on vegetables and cereals. Such have-not diets have been associated with a decrease in incidence of atherosclerotic deposits studied in hundreds of autopsied cases and apparent freedom from symptoms of atherosclerotic complications during life.

The Cholesterol Study

When the first efforts were made to control the atherosclerotic process by dietary means, there was still much to learn about fat metabolism and cholestrol production, or for that matter about atherosclerosis. Nevertheless, by 1950 most American heart specialists were impressed with the probability that blood cholestrol played a prominent role in the atherosclerotic process. It was not certain that the elevation of the cholesterol in the circulating blood was directly related to the atherosclerosis in the wall of the artery. Some even suggested the high levels of blood cholesterol meant it was not precipitating in the wall of the artery. Most heart specialists, however, took a simple pragmatic view, that if it was cholesterol in the arterial wall which caused the heart attack, it was foolish to add additional cholesterol to the bloodstream. One way this might be prevented would be to avoid ingesting cholesterol. These thoughts gave birth to the low cholesterol diet. It was the hope of many heart specialists that merely by limiting the amount of cholesterol in the diet its deposition in the wall of the artery would be decreased. Since the yolk of the egg contained large amounts of cholesterol it was quickly singled out for elimination from the diet.

The thought that the level of blood cholesterol had a direct relationship to its deposition in the atherosclerotic artery was bolstered by studies in the have-not nations. The Bantus and other Africans, the Asians, the Latin and South Americans who were relatively free of the disease had low blood cholesterol values. The blood cholesterol was lower in women than men.

The question was soon raised, what is the normal value for blood cholesterol? Since most Americans already had atherosclerosis, and there was often no way to tell this from a medical examination, there was no way to obtain normal, disease-free, living individuals in the population who could be studied to provide the answer. To this day, in the sense that normal means not associated with the presence of disease, the proper values for blood cholesterol have not been defined. It is clear, however, that blood cholesterol values have been high in the American population for several decades and appreciably higher than in any other group of people in the world. The methods of measuring the amount of circulating blood cholesterol vary widely. Methods have changed as new techniques have developed. Studies in Holland, within the same laboratory, carried out over a period of thirty years, showed a gradual increase in the values in blood cholesterol for representatives of the Dutch population during that period. As prosperity and rich living improved, the blood cholesterol values increased. In general, it appears that the higher the blood cholesterol over a sustained period of time, the greater will be the likelihood of the complications of atherosclerosis, heart attacks, or strokes, and, conversely, the lower the blood cholesterol level the less likely these complications will occur. The blood cholesterol is low in women, low in young, active, lean men, and low in those people of the world who are free of atherosclerosis.

The efforts to use a low cholesterol diet to prevent atherosclerosis, or to simply lower the blood cholesterol, soon ran into difficulties. Evidence began to accumulate that merely restricting the cholesterol intake in the diet did not significantly lower the blood cholesterol in Americans. Early experimental studies on the ingestion of cholesterol, withholding or administering cholesterol in the diet, proved to be such a failure that the low cholesterol diet fell into disrepute. It was soon apparent that individuals eating foods low in cholesterol but still high in fat continued to have high blood cholesterol levels. This observation was better understood when it was appreciated that the liver was able to synthesize cholesterol—acting as a leveling agent to control the amount in the body and circulating blood.

There were other problems which caused difficulty in the experimental studies. Individuals who were placed on a very low-fat diet and then given selected amounts of cholesterol did not appear to absorb the dietary cholesterol. This led to the belief by some investigators that dietary cholesterol was not absorbed from the intestine anyway. Further investigations of this problem have demonstrated that fat in the diet facilitates the absorption of cholesterol from the intestine. A number of the dietary experiments on cholesterol had used crystalized preparations, which were not absorbed from the intestinal tract in the same manner as the cholesterol naturally occurring in meats or high-fat diets.

The confusion that resulted from these different studies still is not completely dispelled, but more recent studies have demonstrated that dietary cholesterol *is* absorbed from the intestine. In the individual on a low-fat diet containing limited amounts of cholesterol, the addition of cholesterol to the diet will elevate the blood cholesterol. In the light of current knowledge, most researchers are of the opinion that the amount of cholesterol ingested in the diet should be sharply limited. This, of course, would be consistent with the character of the diet of the have-not people.

Low Fat Versus Unsaturated Fat

In the evolution of dietary prevention of atherosclerosis the apparent failure of low cholesterol diets to decrease blood cholesterol levels led logically to experiments with a low-fat diet. Initially, no distinction was made amongst the different types of fat—all fat was significantly reduced. Since cholesterol is from food and bile secretion, and is dependent upon the presence of fat in the intestine for reabsorption, the low-fat diet was effective by this mechanism in certain individuals. There are many attractive features to the low-fat diet. It is easy to have a substantial food intake and still significantly lower the calories, because fat, gram per gram, is the richest source of calories. The necessary limitation of meat products and foods containing large amounts of fat and protein cause the low-fat diets to more nearly resemble the diet of the have-not people. A greater emphasis is necessarily placed upon vegetables, fruit, and cereals. Those individuals who achieved appreciable weight reduction through such dietary management frequently had a dramatic improvement in their circulating blood-fat picture. The weight reduction was often beneficial to individuals who had elevated blood pressure, abnormally high blood sugar levels, as well as high blood fat levels. A skilled cook, armed with a variety of good recipes and knowledge in proper preparation, is able to produce good, palatable meals with a wide variety of food choices, using a low-fat diet.

Because the body is able to synthesize fat and cholesterol from carbohydrates and proteins, the low-fat diet was not universally successful. A review of the have-not's diet led some investigators to suspect that the type of fat might be just as important as how much fat. The people free of atherosclerotic disease ate their fat in the form of vegetable oils. The fat in vegetables and seafood both were of the unsaturated variety. Simply changing the diet from dependence on saturated fats, used in the western industrialized nations, to unsaturated fats, demonstrated a marked decrease in the blood cholesterol level in a large number of subjects. While the exact mechanism is not fully understood, the unsaturated fats resulted in a decrease in circulating blood cholesterol, a decrease in beta-lipoproteins, and consequently an improvement in the cholesterol phospholipid ratio. Continued investigations and refinements of this concept have led to the present thinking that the fat in the diet should be restricted to a reasonable amount, preferably less than thirty per cent of the calories ingested, and a large portion of this should be unsaturated fats. In addition, the cholesterol intake should be limited by avoiding cholesterol-rich foods, such as egg yolks, brains, sweetbreads, liver, oysters, butter, and other foods rich in animal or dairy fat.

Unsaturated fats that have only one location on the carbon chain for missing hydrogen are called *mono-unsaturated fats.* Those fats with numerous missing hydrogen atoms are called *poly-unsaturated fats.* Some of the poly-unsaturated fats are classified as essential fatty acids, since they cannot be manufactured from other products by the human body. In some animals, absence of essential fatty acids results in skin lesions or other manifestations of deficiencies. In man, however, a true deficiency state, in these terms, caused by absence of essential fatty acids has not been established. Nevertheless, most authorities agree that the poly-unsaturated fatty acids are important in developing a non-atherosclerotic diet.

The Carbohydrate Story

While looking for differences between the have-nots and the atherosclerotic cultures, the suspicion grew that the whole story could not be answered on the basis of fat alone—either saturated or unsaturated. The Bantu diet was also low calorie, low protein, and low in refined carbohydrates. Sugar, syrups, jelly, and the host of foods containing refined carbohydrates were almost unknown to these peoples. Their carbohydrate sources were closer to natural products, contained in fresh fruit, vegetables, and unprocessed cereals. The non-atherosclerotic Okinawan people ate natural carbohydrates and starchy foods as opposed to refined carbohydrates. The Yemenite immigrants to Israel present an interesting story. Prior to being incorporated into the industrialized society of modern Israel, they had been relatively free of atherosclerosis, even though their diet had contained large amounts of saturated animal fat from milk, cheese, and meat. As they adopted the Israeli cultural patterns and added large amounts of refined carbohydrates to their diet, atherosclerosis increased markedly. On the surface this was highly incriminating evidence, but it was only part of the story attendant to urbanizing Yemenites. Aside from other cultural influences, the average Yemenite gained approximately twenty pounds. The weight gain could not be attributed to increased muscle mass, but, sadly, was obvious evidence of a sustained positive caloric balance with attendant accumulation of dangerous fat deposits.

There is some evidence that increased concentrated carbohydrates, such as starch, will increase blood cholesterol levels. Such experiments need to be carefully analyzed concerning caloric balance, fat accumulation, and level of activity before any sweeping conclusion can be made. There is no evidence to indicate that concentrated carbohydrates such as those found in honey or maple syrup offer any advantages as compared to plain table sugar in lowering blood cholesterol levels.

Endurance athletes and vigorous young pilots, of thirty to thirty-five years of age, having comparable levels of physical activity, frequently maintain a low blood cholesterol level and a favorable blood lipid profile, despite a normal American high-caloric diet. These individuals handle refined carbohydrates very efficiently with a minimal increase in blood sugar values after drinking sugar water. The pattern for the group is distinctly different from less fit young men of the same age, eating similar diets and living under similar socio-economic conditions. The fit individuals, however, have no dangerous fat deposits. Less than eleven per cent of their body weight is fat. These observations suggest that assessing the role of concentrated carbohydrates or of types of protein in atherosclerosis requires adequate consideration of caloric balance and body fat control.

At present a rational approach to the question of concentrated carbohydrates in the diet is to guard against excesses—by getting most of your carbohydrates from natural unrefined sources. If you need to lose fat cut your calories—by significantly reducing or eliminating concentrated carbohydrates in the diet—until your goal is achieved. Thereafter restrict concentrated carbohydrate intake to a level enabling you to maintain an optimal caloric balance. Obvious sources of concentrated carbohydrates, including candy, dessert, and sugared drinks, should be severely limited.

Does Vitamin C Help?

Far more than in the United States, authorities in the Soviet Union place major emphasis on the importance of vitamin C (ascorbic acid) in preventing or treating atherosclerosis. Animals deficient in vitamin C develop atherosclerotic deposits in arterial walls entirely similar to those seen in the human disease. The degree and extent of the atherosclerotic process is related to the severity and duration of vitamin C deficiencies. Atherosclerosis of vitamin C deficiency origin is reversible. When large amounts of vitamin C are given, the abnormal fat deposits quickly disappear. The larger plaques take longer to dissolve. In certain animals the speed of regression is faster. A rapid resorption is seen in dogs because this animal, on a suitable diet, tends to have a low blood cholesterol level, which enhances rapid regression of the atherosclerotic plaque. If extensive, severe plaque formation has developed, residual scarring and damage of the vessel wall is evident. In less severe cases the vessel wall may return to normal.

The blood vessel walls become fragile in the presence of vitamin C deficiency. The vessel wall ruptures easily and a bleeding tendency occurs. Changes in the small capillaries to the arterial wall and perhaps basic cellular changes in the elastic tissue may decrease the arterial wall's natural ability to transmit fat particles without accumulating excessive deposits. There is some evidence that ascorbic acid may resolve plaques in some human cases. Obviously this is the basis for its use by the Soviets. How significant vitamin C deficiency is in the widespread occurrence of atherosclerosis is speculative, but there is enough evidence that a deficiency can be a factor and that all diets, regardless of restrictions, should and must include adequate amounts of vitamin C.

It should be remembered that vitamin C cannot be stored like fat deposits. It is easily destroyed and the tissue stores must be replenished daily. Factors that destroy vitamin C are important and adequate *daily* vitamin C intake is necessary. It has no known toxic action and any excess intake is rapidly destroyed or lost in the urine.

Is Salt Harmful?

Man and animals all need salt. The body fluids normally contain about the same amount of salt as found in sea water. Loss of salt can be dangerous. The body has wonderful mechanisms for eliminating excess salt or retaining salt if it is needed. Of course, gross excess of salt in the diet could be harmful and this is still under study. Any major salt restriction should be only upon the advice of a wise physician. Certain heart patients with accumulation of excess fluid, patients with high blood pressure, kidney disease, and liver disease may require severe salt restriction or medicine to prevent the accumulation of salt and water. These problems, however, require the judgment of your doctor.

The Changing American Diet

Parallel to the increase of atherosclerotic disease in the United States has been a significant change in the American diet. This change has been in the direction of an increase in the amount of meat and concentrated carbohydrates with a general increase in the amount of calories. A few decades ago there were large segments of the American population who did not have regular refrigeration in their homes. The icehouse in those days provided cakes of ice in the heat of the summer for a modest cooling effect, as opposed to the modern-day icehouse dispensing ice cubes for cocktail parties or picnics. The absence of effective refrigeration greatly curtailed the storage of meat and dairy products. Butter could not be kept too long without becoming rancid. Sweet milk soon became sour. It was difficult to keep large stores of meat, even in the winter months. Many a farmer's small supply of meat was dried and smoked or briny preservatives were injected into the hocks of ham in an attempt to preserve them for a longer period of time. The farmer who butchered his own meat had a problem of storing a large animal carcass over a satisfactory length of time.

Money was not so plentiful, preventing purchases of large quantities of expensive meats in the grocery stores. The result of all these factors meant that the rural American of three decades ago depended, to a much greater extent, on vegetables and cereals for his diet. A large segment of the population still lived on the farm. The summer months were a period particularly devoted to eating fresh fruit, vegetables, and melons, as this was the season of their abundance. The housewives busily canned their stores of vegetables and fruit for the coming winter. The home-canned fruits were not packed in heavy syrup as are the commercial products of today. By the end of the growing season most housewives had a well-stocked cellar full of home-canned beans, peas, corn, peaches, pears, apples, pickles, relishes, and all the provisions for the winter months. The bins were full of potatoes and apples. Squash and pumpkins were bedded down in straw.

The usual habit of the rural people gave a cyclic pattern to poultry raising. A frequent meat dish was chicken. Early spring chicks were the early summer fryers. In the winter months there were roast hens and roast turkeys. The beef on the table was, more often than not, what are now considered cheap cuts. The meat dishes were cooked in such a way as to get the most food with the least meat—relying heavily on stews using assorted vegetables. The animals were raised in a somewhat different manner than those raised for the table in subsequent decades. Many of them were grass-fattened steers, meaning their chief source of food was the summer pasture. Only occasional fancy stock breeders, competing for stock show prizes, fed their animals excessive calories of corn and other rich foods to produce an exceptionally fat animal. The beef, veal, and pork that was available was far leaner than that served today. Butter was frequently an expensive commodity. In rural America it was prepared at infrequent intervals with an old-fashioned churn, then rationed out to provide additional flavoring—not as a major spread. Refrigeration, increased money, and very fat animals produced by pen-feeding, have changed all that.

Today ice cream is readily available to anyone. A few decades ago it was prepared for special occasions such as a Fourth of July celebration, or a Labor Day picnic. It was produced by the laborious cranking of the old homemade freezer—wrapped in sacks and blankets. All of these elements of change have helped to produce an American diet fantastically high in fat content, with a large proportion of it belonging to the saturated fat group. The rise in general affluence of the population has provided luxury items for the many instead of the few. Many individuals we consider to be living in poverty are far from starving by the standards of the non-atherosclerotic people of the have-not nations.

With the advent of the supermarket and the modern mass production, the food industries found new ways to preserve their product longer, as well as to give it a more eye-pleasing appearance. Food substances which contain appreciable amounts of unsaturated fats often became rancid or spoiled. Some products, for example peanut butter, didn't give a proper smooth appearance. Old-fashioned peanut butter allowed the peanut oil to float to the top, while the crushed peanut particles settled to the bottom. The separated peanut butter not only didn't last as long on the shelf but it didn't have the same sales appeal as the smooth, even creamy texture present when it was first prepared. The separation problem was obviated simply by adding additional hydrogen to the unsaturated fat chain. The hydrogenated peanut butter could be easily homogenized into a smooth spread, unlikely to have the oil and solid particles separate out. As a result, what beneficial effects could have been obtained from the unsaturated fats of peanut butter were precluded by modern food processing with an eye toward shelf life and sales appeal. These were new hurdles for the biology of man. Nature had not prepared man's system to cope with this type of alteration in his food products.

Changes in the American Weight

As the American diet changed and further industrialization occurred, the weight pattern of the American population changed too. A few decades ago the principal gain in body weight was in the middle-aged person. When you got to be forty you expected to gain weight. In the middle forties usually, the children had grown up and life was becoming more tranquil. With the changes in life's physiology, the decrease in sex hormone secretion was also implicated as a factor in producing the "middle-aged spread." In more recent years the marked weight gain in the American male has been in his latter twenties. The general picture in America today is that many men are middle-aged in terms of body weight when they are twenty-nine years old. They weigh as much now as their grandfathers weighed in their middle forties. In most instances this is not because of increased muscle mass. It represents excess calorie storage.

The danger period for most American men begins when the wedding march ends. There is less time available for recreational pursuits involving physical activity. The new wife is anxious to prove to her new husband that she is a genius in setting a well-stocked table. In their desire to please each other, the wife overcooks and the husband overeats. The outcome is inevitable. A significant and rapid weight gain usually accompanies the first two years of marriage. The greatest ally of atherosclerosis is a loving wife, uninformed about the hazards of food. Soon the husband is ordering larger trousers or old pants have the waistline let out. When this occurs, the wife should realize at once that she is fattening up her husband for the big kill. She may think that his fat rosy cheeks are handsome or are proof to her mother-in-law that she is able to set a good table, but the invisible fat deposits in the coronary arteries tell the real story. A loving wife who looks forward to spending the rest of her life in partnership with her mate should be far more interested in setting the type of table that will avoid excessive weight gain and prevent the atherosclerotic process.

Occasionally weekly periodicals will state that obesity is not a factor in heart disease. Such statements are only half-truths. If you eliminate from a study all individuals whose obesity has caused elevated blood cholesterol, diabetes, high blood pressure, or abnormal electrocardiograms the remaining unique fat people survive rather well. They are the exceptions. Studies of this type are based on poor statistics of a highly selected group. It is similar to concluding that old age has nothing to do with grey hair, because a selected group of older people are not gray. The truth is that the high risk factors of heart disease, high blood pressure, abnormal blood sugar, high blood cholesterol, and even some electrocardiographic changes can all be corrected in many obese people with adequate reduction of body fat. Insurance statistics show an across-the-board increase in disease and disability correlated with obesity.

How to Tell If You Are Overweight

There is no way to determine how much an overweight individual should weigh. This is only "after-the-fact information"— after the excess fat has been removed. Bathroom scales tell only part of the story. It doesn't matter how little you weigh. If you pick up the skin on the abdomen, around the umbilicus, and flatten the fold of skin out and it is over a half inch thick, there is too much fat present. In individuals of average weight, the skin over the back of the hand is loose with no evidence of underlying deposits. This is the way the skin should be over all of the rest of the body if there are no excess fat deposits. This level of weight is far below that considered normal by most physicians and certainly by loving mothers, loving wives, and food-happy husbands.

There is still a general impression that if you don't have fat stores you are sick. Examination of champion endurance athletes in their young years gives a pretty good indication of the amount of fat stores that should be present in vigorous healthy young men.

On examination of a large number of endurance athletes there is no evidence of appreciable fat stores beneath the skin in the area of the small of the back, on the sides, or around the umbilicus—very little more fat than the skin on the back of the hand. This is a physical characteristic of young men in optimal physical condition. I have observed this year after year in endurance athletes preparing for the Olympics. These individuals come close to what might be considered optimal health. Certainly, they cannot be considered underweight or unhealthy. Many of these individuals weigh almost as much as other men in their age group who are fat. The difference is that their body weight is made up of muscle mass. A 150-pound distance runner seventy inches tall will be all muscle mass. A 150-pound office worker of the same height may have a small muscle mass and large fat stores causing rolls of fat underneath his skin, around the small of his back, around his umbilicus, frequently in the buttocks area and sometimes in the thighs.

These two individuals are in no way comparable. The office worker may be carrying a seventeen to twenty-five per cent fat load for his body. The vigorous young athlete may have less than ten per cent body fat. Using the best tests available, including measuring body fat by radioactive techniques, the vigorous young athletes I have studied almost invariably have less than eleven per cent body fat. Some have only six or seven per cent body fat. By contrast, young Air Force pilots, studied by the same method, usually had close to twenty per cent body fat.

It is often stated that seventeen per cent body fat is ideal. In truth, no one has ever demonstrated that this is a satisfactory level for body fat. This value may as well have been picked out of a hat. Values of this sort are often taken from a statistical distribution indicating the most frequent value, but a statistical distribution of the atherosclerotic population is not very comforting since most of these individuals have disease. More pertinent is the percentage of body fat of the have-not people who are non-atherosclerotic individuals. The Bantu and other African groups and the Asians tend to have very lean bodies. Appreciable fat stores are not found on the seventy-year-old war dancers in Africa. Instead, in almost all of these people you will find no significant evidence of fat deposits around the torso. The skin fits tightly over the back muscles and abdomen. There is no "spare tire" here. Judging from healthy young athletes, Swedish gymnasts, and the percentage of body fat in the populations of the have-not nations, the conclusion is inescapable—ideally, your body weight should be controlled at such a level that no dangerous fat deposits appear. If excess fat deposits are present, the calories in the diet and the level of exercise expended must be adjusted in proper relationship to see that all such fat is removed. The closer you come to this goal the more likely that you will be at your optimal weight.

Achieving an optimal weight is a real struggle. First, there are many emotional and psychological factors for eating. It's a pleasant social habit and has been ingrained in business patterns, as well as social activity. In addition, we still live in a culture that considers ample stores of fat to be physically becoming. Almost everyone has his own idea of what constitutes normal weight. The basis for this opinion is usually not the result of having considered the body weight of athletes, young vigorous healthy individuals, or the characteristics of the have-not people. Even your best friends will make a major effort to thwart your success in achieving a proper diet and body fat control. There is a human tendency to like things as they are. If you are fat, your friends and family have become accustomed to thinking of you as fat, they don't want to think of you as thin. This would cause them to have to reassess their own estimate of you—it might even threaten their relationship with you. A wife sometimes fears that if her obese husband loses weight he may be physically more attractive to other women. Some wives subconsciously feel that a skinny husband is a reflection on their cooking. The fat wife fears that a trim husband may insist that she lose weight too. Almost all uninformed office workers will be only too happy to try to give you their expert advice on what you should weigh and what they think of your efforts to lose weight. There is only one solution to this problem—be informed, know what the circumstances are, and then pay little or no attention to the efforts of your associates. If you want to be like everybody else, you can, but in that group of everybody else one out of two dies from heart disease—sometimes at a surprisingly early age. If a wife wants to make a good impression on how well she takes care of her husband, she should point toward having a husband in good physical condition with strong firm muscles—a man who can wear a bathing suit without revealing evidence of sloppy physical habits or an unbalanced diet-exercise program.

Most men achieve physiological maturity before the age of

twenty-five and women sometimes earlier. The bone structure and muscle mass is usually at its maximum before age twenty-five. Unless one begins a weight-lifting career or other forms of increased physical activity after that age, it is unlikely that there will be any further increase in muscle mass or bone. Weight gain, after achieving physiological maturity, usually means deposits of excess fat. Many American men gain fifty pounds between their early twenties and mid-forties. Women are more conscious of their appearance and as a group tend to control their weight better until middle age. With the usual decrease in physical activity, increasing age is associated with diminished muscle mass. For this reason, unless high levels of physical activity are maintained, one should be losing weight with increasing years rather than gaining weight, if excess fat deposits are to be avoided. Maintaining the same body weight from age twenty-five to forty-five is not good enough, if the composition of the body has changed from muscle to fat. The change in body composition to increased fat is often associated with an expanding waistline even though the scales may show no change in body weight. The changing profile provides ample evidence of impending disaster.

How to Gain Weight and Lose Calories

Too much attention is centered on the weight in pounds. This may be very misleading as far as body composition is concerned, providing a false impression about the amount of calories stored. The bathroom scales should be combined with self-inspection in the mirror, awareness of changes in clothing size, and changes in thickness of skin-folds. A fat person of 150 pounds really has stored more calories than a muscular person of 150 pounds. Excessive concentrations on the bathroom scales as opposed to calorie balance is the real answer to the mystery of how you can gain weight on a reconditioning program. Remember that each gram of protein only represents four calories, and each gram of fat represents nine calories. Two and one quarter pounds of protein represent only one pound of fat. The actual ratio is one pound of body fat to five pounds of muscle, because of the difference in water content. During inactivity there is a decrease in muscle mass. If the weight remains constant there is an increase in fat stores. Body weight should decrease because of the conversion of muscle calories to fat calories.

Raw, lean round of beef with all visible fat removed is composed of seventy-two per cent water. A hundred grams (3.5 ounces) contains only 135 calories with 21.6 grams of protein and 4.7 grams of fat. One hundred grams of raw fat separated from the round contains 696 calories and is composed of 18.7 per cent water, 7.5 grams of protein, and 73.6 grams of fat. Similar comparison of ham and leg of lamb demonstrate that fat tissue contains about five times as many calories as lean muscle. If the non-visible fat could also be removed from the lean muscle, the number of calories in muscle would be even less.

A person beginning an exercise program while religiously restricting calories, may be startled to observe a gain in weight even though the waistline has diminished and the fat deposits underneath the skin seem to be less obvious. If a workout program develops new muscle mass, one should expect to convert one pound of fat to five pounds of muscle. Thus, conversion of fat to protein, even on a calorie-restricted diet, can result in gaining weight. The change in dietary habit with conversion of fat to protein, from such a program, can represent a desirable loss of body calories, even though there is an increase in body weight. No population studies suggest that a large muscle mass in a lean person contributes to atherosclerosis. On the contrary, an individual whose body composition is principally muscle with relatively few fat stores, on the basis of a high level of physical fitness, should be expected to be less susceptible to atherosclerosis than a slender unfit individual with excess fat stores.

It is well to establish the habit of keeping track of your body weight. By regular observation, you can learn a lot about the influence of habit patterns on the body weight. A good technique is to weigh yourself each morning upon arising and each evening when going to bed. By doing this, you will begin to appreciate the weight fluctuation associated with daily activity. By taking note of what you eat and what you drink, you will become more aware of the changes in fluid balance that are unrelated to fat gain as well as what dietary factors are associated with your weight changes. A progressive increase in weight without a change in physical activity should warn you to either decrease your caloric intake or increase your level of exercise.

What Diet Should You Use?

In deciding what you should eat, you should first establish your goals. If your weight is stable and you have no evidence of dangerous fat deposits, there need be little concern about caloric intake as long as this situation prevails. The bathroom scales, your clothing, physical profile, and thickness of the skinfold will tell you if you are eating too many calories in proportion to your daily level of physical activity. To lose weight, one should restrict the total amount of fat intake by placing a greater emphasis on vegetables, fruits, and bulk salads—particularly avoiding high-calorie sweets, specifically sugar, syrups, preserves, honey, and molasses. Artificial sweetening can be substituted in most recipes thereby significantly reducing the number of calories available from free sugars. If you do your own baking you can substitute artificial sweetening for sugar. The taste won't be quite the same but the decrease in calories will justify the difference. When artificial sweeteners are used in moderation they produce no harmful effects. Excessive amounts of the artificial sweetener *cyclamate* may induce softening of the stools or diarrhea, and also contribute to increased intestinal contractions due to the laxative effect. In rare cases a large amount of cyclamate can cause an increased sensitivity to sunlight.

The daily consumption of cyclamate should be limited to seventy milligrams per kilogram, or up to five grams for the average adult. In practical terms this means that the daily intake of artificially sweetened soft drinks should be limited to two cans for children and from five to seven cans for adults, depending upon their weight, provided that cyclamate is not used in other foods in the diet. The use of commercial liquid diets—usually four cans a day containing a total of nine hundred calories—is entirely safe from the point of view of artificial sweeteners. But those who consume large amounts of artificially sweetened soft drinks, use the powdered form of artificial sweeteners in their coffee, and then go on a diet using foods also prepared with cyclamate may suffer side effects. However, when one considers that 15,000,000 Americans consume over 80,000 tons of cyclamate annually, it seems that the adverse reactions to cyclamate are extremely rare. The key to the safe use of artificial sweeteners—as for other living patterns—is found in the word "moderation."

In terms of preventing atherosclerosis, the total calories should be restricted to a level which will maintain proper body weight without retention or accumulation of dangerous fat deposits—the visible sign of the invisible killer. The intake of fat in the diet should be limited to a moderate amount, most of which is unsaturated. Sugars and concentrated carbohydrates should be avoided; artificial sweetners are preferred substitutes for sugar. Carbohydrates should come from natural food sources such as vegetables or fruits.

Alcohol has other effects on the heart, which will be discussed later, but *on a weight-reducing diet alcohol has absolutely no place.* Not only does alcohol contribute to the total calorie intake but I have seldom seen an individual who could have one evening cocktail and still control his appetite. The evening cocktail is an invitation to diet failure. While on a restricted diet, if you are attempting to lose excess fat, you should forget alcohol.

While following a significantly restricted diet for purposes of fat loss, you would be well advised to take an adequate amount of vitamins daily. Any of the multivitamin preparations commonly available are adequate for this. If the diet must be prolonged over a period of time, be certain that the vitamin preparation you are using contains some folic acid. Since folic acid is a stimulant to blood formation many vitamin preparations have excluded it.

If for any reason a person should be on a starvation diet (not recommended except under the supervision of a physician), vitamin supplements should be added, since such diets can lead to vitamin depletions. Included should be adequate amounts of thiamine, or the vitamin B complexes, vitamin C, and folic acid. Deficiencies of the vitamin B complexes, if prolonged, can be damaging to the heart, central nervous system, and general body function. Deficiencies in vitamin C have already been mentioned, but in their full-blown form they can cause *scurvy* producing multiple complaints and atherosclerosis.

Food Preparation

Many of the problems associated with a satisfactory diet can be solved in the kitchen. It can truly be said that the first line of defense against atherosclerosis is in the kitchen. Heavy meat dishes, fried in saturated fat, and any other foods fried in deep animal fat are the chief offenders. The best approach is to avoid the frying pan if at all possible. Place a much greater emphasis on food that is roasted, baked, broiled, or boiled. Roasted foods can be permitted to let their fat drip away during cooking, thereby decreasing the residual amounts of fat in the food that goes to the table. In terms of broiling and roasting, you can think of yourself as primitive man roasting his meat on a stake over a flame with the fat products dripping into the fire. Obviously, there is no place in either roasting or broiling for dripping additional fat over the meat. Sauces highly seasoned with onion, garlic, and various spices suitable to individual tastes will go a long way towards improving the tastiness of the meat without adding additional fat. Lemon may be used on fish.

The moisture and flavor of seafood may be maintained by wrapping the fish tightly in foil for baking. If you roast or bake frequently, you can save the drippings from the roast and set them in the refrigerator so that the fat congeals at the top of the container. The fat may then be removed easily and the residual juices used for subsequent baking or roasting. The roasting process need not be accomplished all at one time. Early in the day, the roast may be cooked for about half of its cooking time, then the drippings can be removed, placed in the refrigerator, and the fat separated from the remaining juices. The roasting process may then be continued using the additional juices to baste the meat. Part of the fat-free juices may be saved to make a relatively fat-free gravy.

Although boiled food has become less and less popular in the American diet, boiling meat is one way to eliminate fat. Boiling can be continued until the food is cooked and then set in the refrigerator. The congealed fat which rises to the surface can be removed and the boiled food reheated to the desired temperature for serving.

If you must fry food, use only unsaturated fats for this purpose. Since for the most part the liquid fats usually can be heated to a higher temperature without burning, in this sense, they are better for cooking. Wherever food preparation calls for the use of shortening or fat, use unsaturated fat. If a teaspoonful of lard is called for, use a teaspoonful of cooking oil.

If you are watching calories use artificial sweetener wherever sugar is called for.

Vegetables, Fruits, Melons, and Cereals

Learn to use vegetables, fruits, melons, and cereals as the main source of nutrition. They are remarkably rich in vitamins. Some of these, such as beans and peas, have large amounts of protein. The only precaution that needs to be taken in this regard is to avoid avocados. They are rich in calories and contain large amounts of mono-unsaturated and saturated fats and are relatively poor in the poly-unsaturated fats. Olives and olive oil contain an equal amount of saturated and unsaturated fats. They are not considered beneficial and for the most part should be avoided; they should be considered as a relatively neutral food insofar as saturated versus unsaturated fats are concerned.

Bananas are a fine fruit and as long as one is not concerned about calorie restriction they constitute a good food source. They are exceptionally rich in calories. If it is necessary for you to restrict your caloric intake you should consider this point. For purposes of calorie restriction a greater emphasis should be placed on fruits and leafy vegetables, with lesser emphasis on potatoes, beans, peas, and corn. The potato, either Irish or sweet, is an excellent food source; the skin of the potato is rich in vitamin B complexes. The only valid reason for avoiding it is a necessity to restrict calorie intake. If you don't need to lose fat you may eat potatoes.

Whenever possible use fresh fruit and vegetables. Watch out for canned fruits—many have been packed in heavy syrup. Frozen foods are also often packed with sugar. Most diet food sections have fruit packed in artificial syrup—avoiding an excess of concentrated carbohydrates. Fruits packed in their natural juices are preferable.

Shortening and Cooking Fat

Lard and most solid shortenings shouldn't be allowed in the kitchen. The only shortening or cooking fats that should be used are cooking oils. The best oils, in terms of poly-unsaturated fat content, are safflower oil and corn oil in that order. Soybean oil, peanut oil, and cottonseed oil are far less satisfactory, as they contain larger amounts of saturated fats. Coconut oil is almost exclusively composed of saturated fats and should not be used at all. Olive oil is relatively neutral, but if there is a choice one should use safflower oil or corn oil. For oily salad dressings, mix your own, using as a base safflower oil or corn oil rather than olive oil. The ready-mix commercial low-calorie salad dressings can be mixed with safflower oil or corn oil to provide a favorable proportion of poly-unsaturated fats.

Dairy Products

Whole cow's milk is a rich source of saturated fats and should be avoided. The safest form of available milk is dried, nonfat skim milk. At first, the taste may seem unpleasant but tastes are cultivated. After utilizing these products for a period of time, ordinary whole milk will be foreign to your taste; you may come to prefer the dried nonfat milk flavor. Nonfat dried milk can be used for all forms of cooking or wherever the recipe calls for milk. It provides a good source for protein. The powder may also be utilized in coffee— if one insists on drinking coffee and is accustomed to using cream. Obviously, cream and butter should be avoided. The proper substitute for butter is one of the commercial margarines. These vary extensively; those composed of vegetable oils that have been hydrogenated are no better in terms of saturated fat content than ordinary dairy butter. Other margarines are made with high concentrations of soybean and cottonseed oils. The most satisfactory margarines are those made principally from safflower or corn oil. Unfortunately, it is not possible from the labels on most commercially prepared food to determine how much of the naturally occurring poly-unsaturated fats have been hydrogenated and thereby lose their effectiveness. The labels of most of these margarines indicate that partial hydrogenation has been done. Usually the more creamy the product or the less solid it is at room temperature, the higher will be the concentration of unsaturated fats. Some new butter substitutes are relatively low in calories and saturated fats, containing a reasonable amount of liquid safflower oil and only three and a half calories per gram.

Interestingly enough, most of the fat in cow's milk is saturated. Even though the cow is a strict vegetarian, the bacterial flora in her specialized digestive tract produce saturated fats, most of which are secreted in the milk. A woman's breast milk contains far less saturated fat. In these days of bottle-fed babies this is an interesting observation.

Almost all cheese must be avoided. The "slim cheese"—cottage cheese made from skim milk—is essentially fat-free. It can be used for developing cheese spreads (for example, whipping and blending the cheese with chives or other seasonings) or may be served with sliced tomatoes or fruit when cheese is required in diet preparation. Creamed cottage cheese is to be avoided. Almost all solid cheeses contain large amounts of fat.

The only part of the egg which must be scrupulously avoided is the yolk. Each time an egg yolk is used it should be considered as a large source of both cholesterol and fat. For the most part, the egg yolk should be relegated to the garbage disposal. The white of the egg may be utilized freely as a good protein source. It is essentially free of fat or cholesterol.

Meat, Fish, and Poultry

Fish are your greatest ally. Not only are they relatively low in calories compared to other meats, but almost all of their fat content is of the unsaturated variety. Boil it, bake it, broil it, and—if you must—fry it. Either freshwater or sea fish is a valuable source of protein in the diet. The fat content varies in different fish. Salmon contains a fairly large amount of unsaturated fat. Of the salmon group, chum and pink, or humpback, contain the least amount of fat whereas chinook, or king, and sockeye, or red, are relatively high in fat content.

Sardines contain a relatively large amount of fats, even if packed in tomato or mustard sauce. They should be used sparingly in order to keep the dietary fat intake at a moderate level. If sardines packed in oil are used, it is preferable to find those that are packed in soybean or cottonseed oil rather than olive oil. Mackerel, herring, and eel are relatively high in fat content. Halibut has a moderate amount of fat. Tuna, unless specially prepared, contains excessive fat and is frequently packed in oil. The dietetic-type tuna packed in water is very low in fat. Swordfish, perch, flounder, croaker, bluefish, bass, cod, and trout are relatively low in fat content. Frog legs are exceptionally free of fat and are a good protein source.

Most shellfish, including crab, lobster, shrimp, oysters, and scallops, are relatively low in fat, although they contain an appreciable amount of cholesterol. They can be utilized as low-fat sources of moderate cholesterol content. A three-and-a-half-ounce serving of lobster contains about half as much cholesterol as should be allowed in the daily diet, and a three-and-a-half-ounce serving of oysters contains even more cholesterol than lobster.

Poultry is the other ally to the cook. As a meat source, it contains far less fat than either beef or pork. Free-ranging chickens or those that are not cooped up and battery fed are more apt to have less total fat in their carcass with a higher proportion of unsaturated fat. Young fryers, used for broiling purposes, make a good source of meat which is reasonably low in fat content. Of the different portions of the chicken, the breast and white meat are the lowest in fat content. The dark meat contains a little bit more fat. The skin of the carcass is often rich in fat products; however, part of this is of the unsaturated type. In general, hens of all types of poultry contain a higher percentage of fat than the male. Turkey toms have more breast meat and contain less fat than hen turkeys. Roasting a turkey tom by allowing the fat to drip off the roast into the pan, then avoiding eating the skin, provides a rich source of protein which is relatively low in fat content.

Ducks and geese are loaded with fat—they should be avoided. Wild duck is appreciably better in this regard than the domesticated fowl. The guinea hen, pheasant, and quail are satisfactory sources of meat, whereas squab meat should be considered as equivalent to beef.

Lean beef and veal should be used in limited amounts. A three-and-a-half-ounce serving three or four times a week is really adequate. Although the diet plan recommended by the American Heart Association (see Appendix) includes veal, it should be used moderately. A three-and-a-half-ounce edible portion of veal chuck has an average of ten grams of fat, and half of this is of the saturated type. A similar portion of rib of veal contains fourteen grams of fat, half of the saturated variety. In contrast, a three-and-a-half-ounce edible serving of chicken fryer averages only 4.9 grams of fat, only two of which are saturated. There is a great deal of hidden fat in what appears to be lean beef. This fat is interspersed among the meat fibers and is not visible. All external visible fat should be trimmed off before the meat is cooked. When purchasing meat an effort should be made to buy those cuts that contain the least fat. *Whatever fat comes home with the meat must come off in the kitchen.*

Lean lamb may be utilized sparingly, but excessively fat lamb chops should be avoided. Interestingly enough, goat meat, which is used in some sections of the United States and extensively in Mexico, does not possess nearly as much fat as the domesticated beef animal. It is more comparable to poultry. Venison and antelope are similarly low in fat and comparable to the poultry group.

Pork in all forms should be avoided, including ham, pork chops, and bacon. Under present methods of producing pork, these very fat animals are frequently loaded with saturated fat. A possible exception to the rule of avoiding pork may be made for boiled pork, provided the boiled pork is allowed to set in the refrigerator, permitting the fat to come to the top for removal, then reheating the boiled meat. Even so, removing the very large amount of fat is difficult or impossible.

Almost all forms of luncheon meats, including bologna or other sandwich-type preparations, should be scrupulously avoided. The only exception to this is turkey or chicken meat used for these purposes. Frankfurters, liverwurst, bologna, pressed ham, and the general spectrum of cold cuts are an invitation to dietary defeat. The cold-cut supper may not require much effort in the kitchen but the arteries pay the penalty for laziness.

Desserts

Almost all purchased bakery products are loaded with saturated fats and should be avoided like the plague. *Never purchase cakes, cookies, pies, pasteries, or rolls.* You would be wise to cancel the bakery section from your shopping list. Your avoidance will soon result in a change from unhealthy baking habits to those more compatible with the non-atherosclerotic diet. Bakery products in themselves are not necessarily bad—it's just that most bakeries insist on using saturated fats. The same is true for prepared "slice and bake" products for cookies and a large number of prepared mixes. *Unless you can find on the saleable item clear-cut definite evidence that the preparation has been made with poly-unsaturated fats, which have not been hydrogenated, you shouldn't buy it.* If you don't know what you are buying you are not a wise shopper. Don't be fooled into buying saturated fats through lack of information. The safest approach to cookies, cakes, and pies is to do your baking at home, substituting cooking oils for the usual requested shortening. If a recipe calls for eggs, try it using only egg whites. In many instances, the egg that's included in recipes is not necessary, particularly the yolk. If you want relatively low-calorie baked products, use artificial sweetening as well. A cake prepared with artificial sweetening and poly-unsaturated fats will not be a dietary disaster.

Occasionally you can find a low-calorie cake mix. They are usually low in fat content and suitable for baking purposes. In baking it is well to remember that chocolate, cocoa, and coconut are all rich in saturated fats and should be used in moderation.

Many of the commercial puddings are reasonably low in fat content. Unflavored gelatin is a good protein source without fats or carbohydrates. It is very useful in preparing puddings and fruit gels, or as an added protein source. Cornstarch is a good nonfat additive for puddings or when thickening or smooth texture is desired. Don't forget that fresh fruit makes a good dessert.

Although at one time ice cream was considered a luxury in the American diet, now its exclusion is considered a near disaster by some. Actually, commercial ice cream has less fat in it than some of the old-fashioned homemade ice cream. Commercial producers have learned to increase the size of their products by pumping air into the ice cream to give it a smoother consistency. Some are not adverse to using gelatin products in their preparations for the same purpose. There is such a thing as low-calorie or diet ice cream. The low calorie depends upon whose standards you are using, and you will find that most of these substances do contain an appreciable amount of fat, frequently of the saturated type. You might learn to make your own ice cream. It will require some experimenting, but use the dried nonfat skim milk, add some egg whites and flavoring of your choice. Use artificial sweetening, or if your calorie balance can afford it try honey for a different taste—but remember it is concentrated carbohydrate. Dissolve some unflavored gelatin in boiling water and add it to the mixture. Including some fresh fruit into the mixture helps. You can concoct a delicious, essentially fat-free ice cream in this manner. The types of fruit and infinite flavorings that are available should provide an ample variety. If you want a creamier product without saturated fats and are not concerned about calories, you can add safflower oil to the mix.

If you use an ice tray for the mixture you should put the nearly frozen mixture in a blender to provide a smoother texture. A home ice-cream freezer with regular stirring gives superior results.

Don't forget that frozen dishes can be made of ready-mixed, low-calorie dietary preparations. Read the labels carefully, since some contain sugar and eggs.

Breads

Bread contains an appreciable number of calories and will quickly use up the number that you should be permitted in a day, unless you are engaged in strenuous physical activity. In general, dinner rolls, french bread, and corn bread are relatively high in fat. White, whole wheat, cracked wheat, rye, raisin, and Italian bread may be used without significantly affecting the fat intake. Melba toast, made from any of these, has a relatively low fat content. Most biscuits have even a higher fat content than dinner rolls and should be limited only to occasional inclusion in the diet, and then only if the caloric balance is under proper control. You can bake your own breads, using safflower or corn oils. The "Diet Food" shelf often has low calorie bread products—sometimes without saturated fats.

Soups

Almost all soups can be permitted as long as they do not contain a large amount of fat. A good way to avoid this problem again is to use the refrigerator trick. Cook the soup, let it set in the refrigerator, then skim off the fat from the top and reheat it for serving. If you are preparing a soup that requires the addition of milk, use the nonfat dried milk as your source.

Salads

The appetite can often be satisfied with a good salad. Here is one place where unsaturated fats can easily be added to the diet. Do not use cheese dressings or olive oil. You can mix your own dressings using vinegar or lemon juice and safflower or corn oil. Low-calorie, low-fat mixes are available. The dehydrated packages of seasonings may be used. You can add these to poly-unsaturated oils. Italian and other salad dressings can be mixed half-and-half with corn oil or safflower oil to insure an appropriate ratio of poly-unsaturated fats in the mixture. A large tasty salad will decrease the need for a large meat serving.

A favorite low-fat salad is low-calorie (not creamed) cottage cheese served with fruit or tomato. A low-calorie salad should limit the oil or fat content. Excesses of any food, including salads, can produce fat deposits. It is well to remember that a cow gets "grass fat" on grass alone.

Syrups

Almost all syrups, unless they have been dietetically prepared, contain a large amount of calories. If you must have syrup, you might try one of the low-calorie syrups from the dietetic food shelf in the supermarket. Artificially sweetened preserves may be used in place of syrup on biscuits, pancakes, or toast. There are many artificially sweetened jellies, jams, and preserves—check the diet food section of your supermarket.

Beverages

Regarding their food content, the important consideration of beverages is calories, concentrated carbohydrates, and saturated fats. Large amounts of sugar in coffee, tea, lemonade, or other fruit juices should be avoided. You can use artificial sweetener or omit it. Cream in coffee should be replaced with nonfat milk. A tasty cup of chocolate often contains concentrated carbohydrates, saturated fats, and too many calories. Try nonfat milk and artificial sweetener. The best and healthiest drink is natural fruit juice. The office coffee drinker could do well to drink a glass of orange juice or tomato juice instead of coffee.

Low-calorie diet drinks are preferred to sweetened soft drinks, but excessive use of artificially sweetened drinks should be avoided, as it may cause digestive disturbances. Alcoholic beverages are for social occasions in limited amounts for those not too fat for the calories.

Nuts and Party Snacks

Most tidbits have enough calories for a complete meal. Munching three-and-a-half-ounces of pecans will provide nearly seven hundred calories. A similar amount of peanuts contains nearly six hundred calories. Cheese spreads, cheese bits, fat- or cheese-soaked crackers of all varieties, potato chips, and luncheon meats usually are high in saturated fats and high in calories. These diet pitfalls must be completely avoided.

You can provide healthy snacks. Use cottage cheese made from skim milk and mix it into your own favorite spreads with chives, pimentos, tomatoes, or other favorites. For snacks high in unsaturated fats and low in animal fats use salmon or sardines packed in soybean oil, cottonseed oil, mustard or tomato sauce. Shrimp and crab are delightful and the fat content is low. Some of the "bite-size" cereals of shredded wheat or similar products make a good base for sardines or shrimp as opposed to butter crackers. A plain soda cracker contains five times as much fat as rye wafers and it is all saturated fat.

Don't neglect vegetables for snacks. Cocktail tomatoes, pickles, cauliflower, and "rabbit food" are nonfat with limited calories—a much better prelude to a meal worth eating.

If you must have potato chips—accept the fact that you will get a lot of calories. If you want your fat calories unsaturated make your own potato chips—using safflower oil or corn oil—or be certain the commercial brand has been prepared in unsaturated fat. A better choice is old-fashioned popcorn—popped in a small amount of oil. If you insist on buttered popcorn and don't need to watch calories—pour a small amount of barely melted poly-unsaturated margarine over the popped corn and serve.

Many nuts contain excesses of saturated and mono-unsaturated fats—specifically peanuts and cashews. All nuts are small calorie bombs. Pecans, walnuts, and almonds have a fairly high content of unsaturated fats and are the preferable nuts. An example of the nut problem is the coconut. People using the coconut as a major diet component have extensive atherosclerosis. Coconut oil is chiefly saturated fat and should be avoided. Some people like sunflower seeds which are rich in unsaturated fat but, like all nuts, are rich in calories.

What If You Have an Ulcer?

Many ulcer diets contain a caloric excess and large amounts of saturated fats. Ulcer management is really directed toward neutralizing excess stomach acid. Nonfat milk is just as useful and, if fat is needed, poly-unsaturated oils can be added. Medication for neutralizing acid and relieving spasms are major aids used by the physician. In short: "No, you do not have to eat a high saturated-fat diet if you have an ulcer."

The Breakfast Dilemma

Most of the world is unaccustomed to a large breakfast. The cultural aspects of the American society have been particularly successful in selling the people on the necessity of a large breakfast. The United States, more than any other nation, is the place where a heavy breakfast of eggs, bacon, ham, and other fat-laden products are considered an absolute necessity to begin the day. The silent killer gets an early start, frequently supported by well-meaning dietitians and teachers who are less well-informed concerning the nature of the silent killer or its worldwide distribution. The continental breakfast, limited to a cup of hot coffee, a small unsweetened roll, and fruit preserves, has had no visible deleterious effect upon the daily performance or health of the European. Vast numbers of people in the have-not nations do not have a big breakfast, yet their daily level of activity is unimpaired and in terms of atherosclerosis they are in far better health than the overfed American.

If one is accustomed to eating breakfast regularly and then suddenly stops the habit, initially he will feel exceptionally hungry in the midmorning or he may feel weak or faint. These adjustments are temporary; the body has become adjusted to expecting to be fed on arising and is merely giving a conditioned response. In the healthy individual, a significant curtailment of the breakfast intake for several days will result in a normal readjustment of the body—the undesirable reactions will no longer occur.

If you wish to have breakfast, it should be planned in such a way as to avoid an intake of saturated fats. Any of the cereals may be used, from those commercially prepared to home-cooked oatmeal and rice. If you are accustomed to using cream on your cereal, learn to use a dried nonfat milk preparation. The flavor can be improved by adding fruit to the bowl. If you want coffee and toast, and can't stand dry toast, use safflower or corn-oil margarine. Under no circumstances use bakery-prepared sweet rolls, Danish rolls, or other common products used for breakfast. Breakfast is a good time for fruit juice, fresh fruits, or melon.

Low-fat pancakes can be prepared more easily than dangerous pancakes. Many commercial pancake mixes call for the addition of milk and egg. Neither one of these ingredients is necessary. You can mix an equal amount of pancake mix and water, beat it up, and fry very tasty pancakes, completely free of milk or eggs. You can use nonfat dried milk for better results. Try it both ways. The pancakes can be spread with low-calorie safflower or corn-oil margarine, a low-calorie syrup, or strawberries, preserves, or jellies prepared with artificial sweetener.

How to Find Good Recipes

Changing to a moderate, highly unsaturated fat diet will require some ingenuity and experimenting, which can provide an opportunity for some fun in the kitchen. Chinese and Japanese cooking includes an ample number of tasty dishes, based mostly on vegetables and unsaturated fat. Of course, you should avoid using forbidden meats, specifically sweet and sour pork or excessive amounts of beef. This still leaves a large variety of dishes that are quite satisfactory for a moderate unsaturated fat diet.

The standard American cookbooks are heavily directed toward the use of saturated fats and high caloric foods. Just substitute unsaturated fats in all the places that call for shortening. Try the same recipe without egg yolks, use nonfat milk wherever milk is called for, and use artificial sweeteners. You will be surprised how many tasty dishes can be prepared in this manner, enabling one to continue to eat a satisfying amount of food without danger of accumulating dangerous fat. Cooking in this way, you can develop your own individual dishes. Don't forget to take ample advantage of the different spices. They can perk up an otherwise tasteless dish.

Since the silent killer begins its dirty work early in life, a good dietary program cannot be started too soon. Such a menu is satisfactory for the whole family and can be a means of establishing lifelong dietary habits that are more apt to prevent the ravages, heartaches, and financial disaster of atherosclerosis. Developing a family taste for fresh fruits and vegetables is a major insurance policy toward continued family happiness. The lives of the husbands and sons are literally in the hands of the wives and mothers. The old American kitchen habits have been the first line of defeat in the rising victory of the silent killer. A greater effort in the kitchen will lead to less frustration at the table and less need for excessive willpower or restraint.

An Optimal Diet

There are many opinions and different people have various goals for a diet. The American Heart Association has recommended a diet that meets many of these goals (see Appendix). As a rule, in the light of current knowledge, your diet should include:

1. Less than seventy-five grams (two and two thirds ounces) of fat daily—equivalent to about three and a half ounces of beef fat or a little less butter—with at least half of the fat intake of the poly-unsaturated variety.
2. Less than 450 milligrams of cholesterol daily (see Table on page 125).
3. Adequate vitamin C and other vitamins.
4. More than seventy grams (two and a half ounces) of protein daily—equivalent to the protein contained in eleven and a half ounces of raw lean round steak—(unless you are on a special diet, such as a rice diet prescribed by a physician).
5. Caloric balance adjusted to remove or prevent accumulation of dangerous fat deposits.

These recommendations do not require you to count calories. If you have a fat problem as judged by changes observed in the mirror or the scales and the way your clothes fit, you have to eat less and exercise more to reverse the problem. Counting calories won't help. If you are not controlling or reversing the fat deposit problem, you are eating too much and exercising too little regardless of your calorie bookkeeping.*

The following is a tabulation of the cholesterol content in milligrams contained in one hundred grams (three and a half ounces) of common foods as listed in the U.S. Department of Agriculture's handbook on composition of foods:

* If you want to know more about actual calories and food compositions get *Food Values of Portions Commonly Used,* Church, C. F., and Church, N.H., J.B. Lippincott Company, Philadelphia, 1963, or *Composition of Foods, Raw, Processed, Prepared,* U. S. Department of Agriculture, Agriculture Handbook No. 8, Washington, D.C., 1950, available for $1.50 from the Superintendent of Documents, U. S. Government Printing Office, Washington, D. C. The grams of fat, protein, and carbohydrate contained in various food portions is provided in these books.

	milligrams
Beef, raw	70
Brains, raw	> 2000
Butter	250
Caviar or fish roe	> 300
Cheddar cheese	100
Creamed cottage cheese	15
Cream cheese	120
Cheese spread	65
Chicken, raw	60
Crab	125
Egg whole	550
Egg white	0
Egg yolk, fresh	1500
Egg yolk, frozen	1280
Egg yolk, dried	2950
Fish fillet	70
Heart, raw	150
Ice cream	45
Kidney, raw	375
Lamb, raw	70
Lard and animal fat	95
Liver, raw	300
Lobster meat	200
Margarine, vegetable fat	0
Margarine, 2/3 animal fat	65
Milk, whole	11
Milk, skim	3
Mutton	65
Oysters	> 200
Pork	70
Shrimp	125
Sweetbreads	250
Veal	90

Facts and Frauds in Fat Loss

There is considerable propaganda concerning rapid methods of weight reduction. Most of these methods induce weight reduction without fat loss. The body weight is composed of fat, protein, carbohydrate, bone, and a large amount of water. Then, of course, there is the fully loaded intestinal tract which contributes to body weight. The relatively carbohydrate-free diet, without restriction on meat or fat, results in water loss and not fat loss, unless the calories *are* restricted. In the absence of sufficient carbohydrates, the kidneys tend to excrete larger amounts of salt with an appreciable amount of body water. It is easy to lose five or six pounds of water in a very short time on a low-carbohydrate diet. Unless the total calories have been sufficiently restricted at the same time, this will have no effect whatever on the loss of fat and the body weight will be quickly regained as soon as an adequate amount of carbohydrates are restored to the diet. Such diets can cause great harm and actually can be an ally to the silent killer.

The indiscriminate ingestion of large amounts of protein, containing with it large amounts of saturated fats, can only lead to a rise in the beta-lipoproteins in the circulating blood volume with a consequent increase in their migration through the arterial wall and subsequent atherosclerosis. In addition, such diets are deficient in fruits and vegetables that contain naturally occurring vitamin C, which may significantly contribute to the integrity of the arterial wall. You should not succumb to such recommendations. There is no easy shortcut to fat loss that can give you instantaneous crash results that should be used without close supervision of a knowledgeable physician.

Bed rest, as explained in relationship to environment, can cause a rapid loss of water. Even in normal healthy individuals without excessive stores of fat, the loss of water can represent a weight loss of four to six pounds. This is not fat loss but is directly related to the body's horizontal position and is quickly regained as soon as normal living activities are resumed. Weight loss of this type has no beneficial physiological effect whatever. Water emersion has an effect similar to bed rest, in that it compresses the external venous reservoir and increases the return of blood to the heart. Prolonged emersion causes a rapid loss of body water which can lead to faintness and weakness. The water loss is temporary. Whirlpools, water massages, and water baths should all be considered as inappropriate methods for weight reduction. Whirlpools and physiotherapy have an important place in the management of muscle disorders or in other medical problems, but they have no place in fat reduction. The same may be said for heat, steam baths, or the recent fad— sauna baths. The only easy shortcut is in the kitchen, and that is through proper food preparation.

The Wonder Pill

A variety of pills have been advised and used in an effort to prevent atherosclerosis or in an effort to induce fat loss. Some of these are complete frauds while others are beneficial. Those prescribed by intelligent bona fide physicians are often of great use and even essential to health. Those prescribed by non-physicians and passed out by quacks may be dangerous to the point of causing death.

Some individuals require thyroid pills because their thyroid gland is functioning at an abnormally low rate. The medication is indicated because of the low thyroid function and not necessarily because of the increased weight. The adequate administration of thyroid under these circumstances commonly results in satisfactory fat loss with a decrease in the level of circulating blood cholesterol and beta-lipoproteins. There is no harm in the correct administration of thyroid replacement.

Some patients need medications that cause the kidney to excrete water. These medications are used only when an abnormal retention of water has occurred in the body, such as in the presence of kidney or heart disease. They are sometimes used in women who accumulate excessively large amounts of fluid just preceding the menses. The proper use of such medications prevents the tension, headaches, and other discomforts associated with this problem. Again, this is a straightforward medical indication and not intended as a method of fat reduction.

Some physicians use an appetite suppressant pill, at least for an initial period, in individuals who have difficulty in controlling their diet. Its use is on less firm ground and of course not usually employed in individuals who have significant evidence of abnormal heart or circulatory function. They can, however, be used under a qualified physician's supervision in limited cases. The same result can usually be achieved by switching to an adequate bulk, low-calorie diet of the type which can be easily developed from the principles outlined in this chapter.

There have been, and will continue to be, testings of various pills that can be used to lower blood cholesterol or beta-lipoprotein levels. Some of these act to prevent the absorption of fats in the intestine; others have a more complex biochemical action. Some medications may one day prove to be as important in the problems of handling fat as insulin has proved to be in the problems of handling carbohydrates in the diabetic. Minimal success has been reported with some of these preparations. None of them yet have proved to be sufficiently effective over a long period of time, without harmful effects, to be used on a wholesale basis. In short, there is no wonder pill for lowering the blood fat level that can accomplish for you today what can be accomplished in the kitchen.

Finally, there are the quacks and frauds who distribute a wide variety of medications indiscriminately to patients who wish to lose weight. These are usually not given by certified, licensed medical physicians. Often such pills include appetite suppressants which stimulate the central nervous system and reduce hunger; they may include a substance to cause the kidneys to excrete excessive amounts of water, which will also take with it important salts such as potassium. Some of them contain digitalis, a heart drug which is very useful in heart patients when administered properly. When it is given indiscriminately, particularly in the presence of a medication to cause loss of body water and salts, this medication can cause major abnormalities in the function of the heart, including death. The lesson to be learned from all of this is—do not take any pills unless they are prescribed by your physician, and know your physician well enough to know his qualifications.

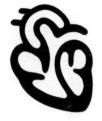

CHAPTER VII

Exercise — Dangers and Benefits

PHYSICAL ACTIVITY if used properly improves the functional capacity of the heart and circulation. The important phrase is "used properly." Similar to many life-saving medicines, *it* can be a killer if used carelessly. Some heart patients should not exercise. Some individuals who have never had a heart attack can cause one by improper exercise. Correctly used, exercise may help to prevent a heart attack or improve your chances of survival, if you have one. The stakes are too high for you to be an uninformed exercise enthusiast. Despite current enthusiasm, it is well to remember that exercise can kill you.

Exercise Helps Control Your Weight

Any increase in physical activity will increase the calories required by the body. Work requires energy, energy requires calories. It does require a lot of work to use the number of calories in one pound of fat. Regular physical activity, however, on an accumulative basis can utilize a large number of calories. To lose a pound of body fat, you must use 3500 calories (some water contributes to the weight of body fat). If you increase physical activity sufficiently to use an additional two hundred calories a day, by the end of a year this would be equivalent to 73,000 calories, or more than twenty pounds of body fat. For most individuals, this represents a daily walk of less than one hour's duration.

The calories used for walking depend upon the speed and weight of the individual. Walking at three miles an hour, an individual weighing a hundred pounds will utilize three calories per minute. A 150-pound person will use four calories per minute, and a two-hundred-pound individual uses a little more than five calories per minute. A 150-pound person, walking three miles an hour, will require 240 calories per hour. If he walks a half hour a day *and does not increase his caloric intake,* he can expect to lose over twelve pounds in one year.

Most people have the same problem in using physical activity to control body weight as they do with diet programs. They want instantaneous results. Like crash diet programs, *crash exercise programs are usually ineffective.* The average individual would have to walk 435 miles to lose ten pounds of body fat; obviously this cannot be done as a crash effort. The required reduction in food intake sounds equally forbidding as a total sum; to lose ten pounds of body fat a person would have to eliminate over fifty pounds of lean meat or ten pounds of meat fat from the diet. The same effect can be achieved by consistently eliminating two and one-half ounces of lean meat (less of ordinary meat) or less than one ounce of carbohydrates, or less than one-half ounce of fat each day from the diet for one year.

The average individual uses twice as many calories during calisthenics as he uses while resting. Playing and practicing football requires the expenditure of an additional 2500 calories a day. Housekeeping usually requires an additional 1600 calories a day, although the variation here can be quite large. Sporadic peak loads of exercise are the real danger. An example of one of these is shoveling snow. Clearing the snow from a wide area can be disastrous for the overfed, underfit individual. Lifting and throwing away one average shovelful of snow can require over two hundred milliliters of oxygen (one calorie of energy) or nearly double if it is wet snow. At this cost, it doesn't take very long to expend a large number of calories and you need to be in tip-top physical condition to pursue this activity over any length of time.

The balance between caloric intake in terms of food and calorie expenditure by physical activity is a major factor in the control of body weight. The best way to determine whether you have the proper balance, if you are trying to lose weight, is to determine if you are losing excess fat deposits. If you have already lost all of your excess fat deposits and are merely interested in preventing the accumulation of fat, testing the thickness of the fat deposits under the skin and around the body is the best guide to determine whether or not you are achieving your objective.

You Need More Oxygen for Work

The metabolism of fats, carbohydrates, and proteins requires varying amounts of oxygen, but on a mixed diet one liter (approximately one quart) of oxygen is required to metabolize enough nutrient material to generate 4.86 calories. For a college football player, using an additional 2500 calories a day for his activities, this would require the circulation to transport an additional five hundred liters of oxygen daily. An increased daily expenditure of only two hundred calories requires the circulation to transport an additional forty liters of oxygen daily. During vigorous exertion in young men, oxygen requirements may reach three to four liters a minute for a short period of time. The additional oxygen needed for increased levels of physical activity must be delivered by the circulation. In this way, exercise influences the action of the heart and circulation.

The Heart Pumps More Blood

One way to increase the transportation of oxygen is to increase the amount of blood pumped by the heart. This is accomplished by increasing the amount of blood the heart pumps with each beat (stroke volume) and increasing the heart rate.

Under normal resting circumstances only about half of the blood is ejected from the right and left ventricular cavities with each heartbeat. As the demands on the heart are increased, the heart simply empties more completely with each beat. The ability to increase stroke volume varies, particularly in relation to the level of physical fitness. In some individuals the increase is minimal and an increased heart rate is the principal way of augmenting cardiac output. Increasing the stroke volume is an economical way to increase cardiac output. Increasing the heart rate is far more expensive. During exertion, endurance athletes in peak condition may have a stroke volume well in excess of 150 ml, twice that observed under normal resting conditions.

The heart rate increases as the level of work increases. The faster the heartbeats, the less time is available for the heart to refill with blood before each contraction. These and other factors related to the mechanical pumping action of the heart limits the stroke volume of each heartbeat. The maximum advantage of the combination of increased heart rate and stroke volume usually occurs at a heart rate of around 180 beats per minute. If the heart rate is too high, the heart becomes less efficient as a pump and the cardiac output falls. Individuals with various forms of heart disease may not be able to tolerate the higher heart rates commonly seen in athletes and young people. Children tolerate higher rates than adults while still increasing the pumping action of the heart. Heart rates of over two hundred beats per minute in youngsters during vigorous exercise are well within the limits of the maximum effectiveness of the healthy young heart.

A young adult male in good physical condition is capable of increasing his heart rate to 180 beats per minute while maintaining a stroke volume of 150 ml per beat, which means that the heart is pumping twenty-seven liters (over twenty-eight quarts) per minute. Values much higher than this can be achieved by endurance athletes. When this figure is compared to an average cardiac output at rest of five liters per minute, one can appreciate the range of function for the pumping action of the heart. This range of function enables the circulation to control the delivery of oxygen as it is needed.

More Oxygen Is Taken out of the Blood

A second way the circulation can increase the delivery of oxygen to the tissues is simply to take more oxygen out of each circulating unit of blood. Since blood returns to the right heart still carrying about seventy per cent of the oxygen it had when leaving the left heart, it is apparent that much more oxygen could be extracted. This reserve capacity is utilized when exertion requires more calories. At the peak of maximum exertion, the oxygen saturation of blood returning to the great right atrium drops to twenty-five per cent. By increasing the oxygen extraction to this degree while increasing the cardiac output to twenty-seven liters, the circulation transports fifteen times as much oxygen during exertion as it transports at rest. This ratio is even greater when the cardiac output is larger. In outstanding endurance athletes the circulation is able to transport more than twenty times as much oxygen during exertion as during resting circumstances.

The more complete extraction of oxygen is accomplished by controlling the blood distribution. The working muscle groups need the increased amount of oxygen so they get the major portion of the increased cardiac output. Most of the increased cardiac output is shunted to the leg muscles during running. The liver, kidney, and abdomen have no need for an increased flow of blood. The work of the kidney as a filter is essentially unchanged. The large percentage of the cardiac output that goes to these areas under resting circumstances is sharply reduced. The actual blood flow to the liver, kidney, and abdominal area during physical exertion is often less than during resting circumstances. The muscles that are not being used during exertion also receive less blood flow. If the arm muscles are not being used during a period of exercise, the blood flow to these muscle groups is diminished while the oxygen extraction from the diminished blood flow is increased. The venous blood returning from the nonworking muscle of the arm will be very low in oxygen content because, although the arm receives less blood, it extracts more oxygen from what it does receive.

To accomplish an efficient distribution of blood during exercise, complex reflex mechanisms must control the size of the various arteries. This is done by relaxing the muscular cuffs located in the vessel wall. If running, walking, or similar exercise is involved the arteries in the legs dilate, while the arteries that supply the abdominal organs and the arms constrict. This is a variable adjustment. The redistribution of the percentage of cardiac output changes gradually as the level of physical activity changes. Considering the vast number of arteries that are affected, the smooth integration of these adjustments on a continuous basis is one of nature's marvels.

The Blood Pressure Goes Up

When the amount of blood pumped into the arterial tree is increased, the pressure in the arteries goes up. There is a fundamental relationship between pressure, blood flow, and resistance offered by the arteries. As the level of exercise increases, the systolic blood pressure increases. Values in excess of 240 mmHg are not uncommon. The rise in pressure is not as great if the terminal arteries to the muscles and distal portions of the circulation relax. A very elastic great aorta can accommodate part of the increased stroke volume by its own expansion. Despite the different factors involved, the usual pattern is a gradual rise in systolic pressure parallel to the increase in physical effort.

The diastolic pressure may rise only slightly or remain unchanged in young, reasonably fit individuals. This is an indication that the distal arteries are relaxed, offering minimal obstruction to blood flow. The difference between the systolic and diastolic pressure (the pulse pressure) may increase enormously during maximum exertion. The rise in pulse pressure tends to parallel the increase in stroke volume.

The Heart Needs More Oxygen

The heart must work harder to pump more blood and, like any other working muscle, uses more energy which requires more oxygen. The blood supply to the heart muscle is unique. As discussed in Chapter III it is the only portion of the circulation where increased oxygen extraction cannot be used to any significant advantage. Even while resting, the venous blood returning from the beating heart muscle contains only about 5 ml of oxygen. *The only way more oxygen can be delivered to the working heart muscle is to increase the blood flow through the coronary arteries.* Blood flows through the coronary arteries to the heart muscle while the heart muscle is relaxed or in diastole. An increased heart rate decreases the time to permit filling of the coronary arteries.

To increase the blood flow to the heart muscle the coronary arteries dilate, just as they do during oxygen deprivation at higher altitudes. The dilated coronary arteries offer less resistance to the flow of blood and more blood flows to the working heart muscle. When this cannot occur, for example, because of atherosclerotic disease of the coronary arteries, the increase in blood flow to the heart muscle will be limited. In this way, advanced coronary artery disease may limit the work the heart muscle can do.

On a temporary basis, the heart may use high-energy compounds that are stored in the heart muscle fibers (see Chapter III). These may be thought of as high-energy fuels (such as creatinine phosphate). The use of these substances to liberate energy does not require oxygen. Their original formation requires oxygen and oxygen is required to replenish them in the heart muscle. These high-energy compounds represent reserve energy stores which can be used in case of an emergency. They enable the heart muscle to develop an oxygen debt—the heart is able to use up various energy stores to achieve its work without oxygen, then rebuild the energy stores later.

How Strong Is Your Heart Muscle?

The effective work of the heart muscle is directly dependent upon the pressure it creates by its contraction and the length of time this pressure is sustained. The heart muscle must work a great deal harder to sustain a systolic pressure at levels above 200 mmHg than it does to sustain a pressure of 120 mmHg. If the higher levels of pressure are repeated at frequent intervals, because of increasing heart rate, the total number of times the heart muscle must contract this forcefully is increased. The work of the heart, then, is closely related to the level of systolic pressure and the heart rate. If the heart rate reaches 180 beats per minute and the systolic pressure is 240 mmHg, the work of the heart muscle is far greater than during rest with a systolic pressure of 110 mmHg and a heart rate of approximately seventy beats per minute. The heart muscle has to develop sufficient strength to work at high levels of activity. The heart muscle is similar to other muscles such as those found in the leg. Weak leg muscles will not permit a person to walk or run a great distance. The limitation of the work capacity for the leg muscles is usually not their blood flow but the strength and physical characteristics of the muscle fibers. Weak muscles mean a weak effort regardless of the available blood supply. The heart's ability to work depends upon the strength and endurance capacity of the heart muscle itself independent of its blood supply. Even though the blood supply to the heart muscle is adequate, if the muscle is weak and flabby, the level of work it can achieve and sustain will be significantly limited.

Steady-State Exercise

Physical activity sustained for an appreciable period of time, usually over six minutes, at a constant level well within the capacity of the circulatory system is called *steady-state exercise.* The heart, lungs, and circulation adjust to the new level of energy requirements at an even constant level. The heart rate stops fluctuating and levels off. The stroke volume for the heart should also level off, thus causing the amount of blood pumped by the heart to remain fairly constant. The adjustments in the different arteries to the distal regions of the body, the level of respiration, and the level of energy expenditures by the different muscle groups, all remain at a fairly constant level. The amount of exercise which can be sustained in a steady state for any appreciable length of time is far below the maximum peak ability of an individual. Some individuals can sustain a very high level of physical activity for hours. Some of the best examples are marathon runners. These well-trained competitors maintain a fairly even level of activity for well over two hours. In terms of developing strength and capacity for the heart and circulation, prolonged periods of exertion in the steady state are perhaps the most beneficial. The heart muscle must be regarded as an endurance muscle. It can be trained only by endurance exercise. This does not mean a high level of activity but a sustained and prolonged effort.

More Arteries for Heart Muscle

When a muscle is exercised adequately for sustained periods of time, the number of blood vessels supplying it is increased. As the number of small capillary vessels increases, the size of some small arteries is enlarged. This is one of the strongest arguments for the use of physical activity in the prevention of heart attacks. The increase in blood supply to the heart muscle has been well documented. Studies have been carried out using rats and guinea pigs swimming to exhaustion in tanks of water. The animals were killed and their arteries were injected with a rubber plastic-like material; then the heart muscle around the vessels was removed. The size and number of the vessels were significantly increased in the animals with an increased level of exercise.

There are abundant specimens of diseased hearts and hearts from invalids, but the opportunity to study the blood vessels to the heart muscle of vigorous athletic individuals seldom occurs. Thus it is hard to demonstrate conclusively in man that exercise increases the blood supply to the heart muscle. This difficulty has been circumvented to some extent by studying the autopsy specimens of individuals with problems that increased the work of the heart muscle. Some examples involved an increased workload for the right ventricular muscle mass and others for the left ventricular muscle mass. These hearts were compared to those from individuals who were dibilitated or at bed rest because of chronic diseases not directly related to the circulation. Although the size of the major arteries to the heart muscle was not always significantly increased, the most striking difference was the increase in the smaller arteries and blood vessels. The connections between the terminal branches of the right and left coronary arteries were markedly increased in number. This is anatomical evidence of the ability to increase the blood supply to the heart muscle, through either the right or the left main coronary artery. At present, there seems to be sufficient evidence to state that *exercise is an important factor in increasing the blood supply to the heart muscle and in improving the number of connections between the major arteries,* thereby improving on nature's redundancy system to supply blood to different regions of the heart muscle through more than one source.

The size and the number of the arteries are very important, since even if there is atherosclerotic disease of the vessel walls, if the arteries are large enough, blood will still get to the heart muscle. When disease of the major arteries results in coronary artery thrombosis, if the other arteries are open and the teminal connections between the two arteries are sufficiently numerous, most of the heart muscle will still get an adequate supply of blood—at least for resting requirements. In this way, the increased vascularity of the heart protects the heart muscle from infarction or death even in the presence of coronary occlusion. This may be the major benefit of exercise—a benefit that can save your life!

The Circulation of the Fit

An individual in peak physical condition is so rare in the American population that an examining physician may suspect him of having heart disease. This is a sad commentary on the level of physical activity for the general American population. Most practicing physicians either see individuals with very average hearts, which means they are not at optimal condition, or else they see individuals with diseased hearts. When a well-conditioned athlete, or an individual otherwise in good peak physical condition, presents himself to a physician, he may be an oddity. Endurance athletes such as the distance runner, the skier, and the swimmer are perhaps the best examples of well-conditioned people.

The well-conditioned man usually has clearly defined muscle patterns and the skeletal muscles of the body are firm, indicating good muscle tone. There is little or no evidence of fat deposits either about the waist or the small of the back. The resting heart rate is the first thing which may alert the examining physician. Many athletic young men have resting heart rates below fifty beats per minute. It is relatively uncommon in today's society to find individuals without heart disease who have resting heart rates between forty and fifty beats per minute. The very slow heart rates seen in these individuals are the direct result of their level of training. This is well illustrated by the changes in heart rate noted in the case of Roger Bannister. Prior to the time he began training to be the first man in history to run the four-minute mile, his resting heart rate was commonly in the mid-seventies. By the time he had improved his physical condition to the point that he was able to establish an historic new record, his resting heart rate was commonly below forty beats per minute.

To observe the slow-resting heart rate of the well-conditioned man, the heart rate must be taken during periods free from tension or excitement. Many an experienced heart specialist has made the mistake of assuming that an endurance athlete's resting heart rate was rapid by studying the heart rate at the wrong time. The excitement of impending competition frequently increases the heart rate of the athlete. Studies taken even days before the anticipated competition reveal an increase in the heart rate. In some instances, just preceding the race, the heart rate may be appreciably more rapid than noted immediately after the race is finished. These apparent discrepancies do not detract from the general observation that well-conditioned individuals have slow resting heart rates. This is true of women as well as men although the heart rates for women in general are a little faster. This correlates well with the difference in body size. Small animals have very rapid heart rates while larger animals usually have slower rates. Elephants, for example, often have heart rates of only thirty beats per minute. The slow rate and increased size of the well-conditioned human heart provide at least some justification for saying that such an individual has "the heart of an elephant."

Mild exercise may not significantly increase the heart rate of persons in peak physical condition. The simple exercise test commonly used in the physician's office—in which the patient takes a number of trips over two steps in a three-minute period—is usually not enough to increase the heart rate very much for these athletes. A person with a resting heart rate of fifty beats per minute or below, often has the same heart rate after the exercise is completed. The level of physical activity required is literally so far below the maximum capability of the circulatory system that the heart is barely stimulated. After a period of relatively heavy exercise of sufficient degree to significantly increase the heart rate of a fit individual, the recovery period is fairly short. The length of time required for the heart rate to return to its pre-exercise level is minimal, compared to that of the unfit individual.

One of the adaptations the heart of an endurance athlete makes is to increase its stroke volume capacity. The heart muscle fibers gradually lengthen, increasing the capacity of the ventricular chambers. The heart size is often larger than seen in similar nonathletic individuals. The apparent increased size of the heart is one of the features which has caused physicians to be suspicious of the so-called "athletic heart." Certain heart diseases are also associated with enlargement of the heart. When the heart muscle fails, the fibers are extended to their absolute length, but the mechanism is entirely different. In the failing heart the muscle fibers are overstretched because they have been too weak to maintain adequate contraction. In the athletic heart the lengthened fibers are a result of normal adaptations, which improve their strength and enable the ventricular cavities to hold and pump more blood.

The increased size of the endurance athlete's heart is partly related to its increased capacity to store blood or increase its stroke volume—in this sense it is dilated. The size of the heart muscle is also increased. Maintaining high levels of systolic pressure during a rapid heart rate for a great length of time requires the heart muscle to work harder. Like all muscles in the body, work changes their characteristics. The heart muscle of the well-conditioned individual is strong, with good tone. It is very flexible to permit maximum internal efficiency during contraction. One can hardly expect an average muscle to accomplish an above-average workload.

In the resting state the blood pressure of the well-conditioned individual is similar to his less fit counterpart, excluding relatively obese individuals. The well-conditioned individuals as a group have lower systolic and diastolic pressures than the average fat person. To the extent that physical training helps to control the body weight, it has a direct relationship to the level of blood pressure.

Physically fit individuals can stand upright and motionless without fainting, or having a significant change in heart rate. Even the fit individual may faint under stress or from emotional stimuli, but the wide variation in heart rates associated with motionless standing in less fit individuals is usually not observed in the well-conditioned individual. Physical fitness also increases the circulating blood volume, which is one of the factors that enables him to stand motionless without significant changes in the circulation. Increased blood volume also helps him to transport large quantities of oxygen during periods of maximum exertion.

The Circulation of the Unfit

The features of the circulation of the unfit individual are just the opposite of those noted in the fit individual. The heart rate may be relatively rapid, even at rest. Usually, the higher the resting heart rate, the less fit the individual. Aside from lack of exercise this can also be caused by tobacco, excessive coffee or tea, alcohol, or anxiety. The unfit individual usually has a small heart with a small stroke volume capacity. Any increase in cardiac output is caused almost exclusively by increasing the heart rate. Mild exercise will increase the heart rate of the unfit individual markedly. If an obese forty-year-old American male does the double-step test, mentioned earlier, immediately after the exercise his heart rate may exceed one hundred beats per minute. Even an older individual in optimal physical condition may have a slow-resting heart rate, unchanged by the same exercise test. As a general observation, if you take your heart rate while lying down after a minimal amount of exercise and find it higher than a hundred beats per minute, the cause should be sought. The first step is to eliminate coffee and cigarettes, and the second is to increase the level of physical activity, unless obvious disease is present.

The blood volume of the unfit individual is relatively small and on standing, the heart rate increases to surprisingly high levels. Studies of the blood supply of bedridden individuals suggest that the number of arteries and interconnections between them, so important in protecting against myocardial infarction, are significantly reduced.

Different Exercises Develop Different Hearts

Maximum exercise of small muscle groups, like the hand muscles, requires little additional oxygen and does not increase the work of the heart very much. Exercise which strengthens the heart and improves the circulation involves large muscle groups. Walking, running, jogging, swimming, bicycling, and skiing all use large muscle groups. Activities of this type place significant demands upon the circulation.

Endurance exercises, such as long distance running, develop the type of heart previously described for the fit individual. Exercise that involves skill, such as throwing the discus or the javelin, does not require great amounts of energy over a sustained period of time and may not condition the heart as an endurance muscle. Short maximum efforts often are not effective in increasing the capacity of the heart or significantly lowering the resting heart rate. The weight lifter's heart is considerably different in configuration and characteristics from the long distance runner's. Usually, it is more nearly the same size as the average individual of similar age and body-type. The resting heart rate is more rapid than in the endurance athlete, and all indications are that the heart is not developed to the level of its maximum capability as an endurance muscle.

What Limits Your Exercise Capacity?

No one factor alone limits anyone's level of exercise. The strength of the muscles in the arms and legs or groups involved in a particular physical activity may be the limiting factor. For example, the amount of exertion you can do with your arm usually is limited by the strength and endurance capacity of the arm muscles. The heart and circulation are normally well equipped to meet any demand required by this type of activity—the limit to the level of exertion is strictly the limit of the functional capacity of the muscles in the arm.

There are several ways in which the heart may be the limiting factor to exercise capacity. Perhaps the most common way is by its limited characteristics as an endurance muscle. A weak heart muscle, unable to sustain repeated vigorous contractions, cannot sustain the high level of action necessary to pump large volumes of blood for any appreciable length of time.

Another factor, balanced against the strength of the heart muscle, is the blood pressure. The heart muscle has to work harder to pump the same amount of blood if the arteries offer major resistance to the ejection of blood by the heart. Even a strong, vigorous muscle may be limited by increased arterial blood pressure. In this way, blood pressure poses a limiting factor on the heart muscle's ability to pump blood and may cause it to reach its maximum capability at a less efficient level.

Inadequate return of venous blood to the heart can limit even a vigorous, healthy heart muscle's pumping action. If there is not enough blood getting back to the heart, it doesn't matter how strong and vigorous the heart muscle is; its ability to pump blood will be limited. Thus, either the arteries or the veins can significantly alter the function of the heart as a pump.

The heart's pumping ability also may be compromised by damaged valves. When the aortic valve at the outlet of the left ventricular cavity is damaged or doesn't close properly, the amount of blood that leaks back into the left ventricular cavity is really lost to circulation. If the left ventricle ejects 150 ml of blood into the great aorta and 50 ml leaks back, the effective stroke volume is only 100 ml. Individuals with disease of the aortic valve develop a large, strong heart muscle, in an effort to compensate for the additional load created by the leaky valve. Even though the heart muscle is strong and vigorous, leaky heart valves can compromise the pumping action of the heart.

Some authorities feel that the major limitation to the heart's ability to pump blood to the lungs and the rest of the body is literally the blood supply to the heart muscle—the coronary blood flow. It is assumed that diseased coronary arteries limit the capacity to provide blood for the working heart muscle and limit the work the muscle can do. This is certainly true in extreme conditions—particularly in advanced coronary artery disease. Tests of several thousand forty-year-old American males to the point of maximum exertion identified only a very small percentage who had any evidence of limited exercise capacity because of limited blood supply to the heart muscle. A more likely cause for exercise limitation in such individuals is the limited strength of the heart muscle itself—a reflection of inadequate regular exercise. Inadequately exercised heart muscle is weak and may have a marginal coronary blood flow system.

The body weight is an important factor in all exercises in which the body weight must be lifted or moved, such as running, tennis, football, or similar activities. Pedaling a stationary bicycle-type device, in which the body weight is totally supported by a seat, is less apt to be influenced by body weight. Pedaling exercises done while lying down also are less apt to be influenced by body weight. In running-type exercises, or walking on a treadmill, body weight definitely limits the distance an individual can go. Using treadmill exercises with a gradually increasing grade of the walk, the more a person weighs the more work he has to do. He will reach his maximum work level in a shorter length of time than a comparable individual who weighs less. Repeated studies of individuals undergoing weight reduction demonstrated improvement. One way, then, to improve the exercise capacity of an individual who is moderately overweight, even though he may have heart disease, is to reduce his body weight. If the ability of the heart to pump blood is unchanged, the decreased body weight will decrease the amount of energy that must be expended for a given task, and therefore the individual can walk longer at steeper grades. Many patients with heart disease can be more active if they lose excess fat.

Usually the lungs do not limit exercise capacity. The amount of air required to provide oxygen for the circulatory system is far below the capacity of the lungs. Chronic lung disease or other abnormalities in the function of the lung may fail to supply an adequate amount of oxygen, therefore lowering the oxygen content of the blood leaving the lungs and increasing the work of the heart.

Anemia, with a decreased number of red blood cells or less hemoglobin per unit of blood, decreases the amount of oxygen each unit of blood carries. This limits the circulation's capacity to deliver oxygen to the tissues and limits the level of exertion.

An overactive thyroid gland can increase the amount of oxygen used by the heart and other tissues at rest. The margin of reserve capacity remaining between the resting requirements and that available for exertion severely limits the level of exercise.

Exercise Alone Does Not Prevent Heart Disease

There is a popular thesis that all one needs to do to prevent heart disease is to exercise adequately. This is particularly comforting to those who like to eat large amounts of rich food, drink, and smoke. While there is no doubt that exercise is beneficial, the simple truth is that it may not prevent coronary atherosclerosis. The concept that exercise prevents heart attacks and significant coronary-artery disease received much support in recent years from the case of a seventy-year-old Boston marathon runner, Clarence De Mar, a superb athlete who remained in tip-top condition until he was stricken with cancer. This unusual circumstance permitted an opportunity to examine the status of his heart and blood vessels. The main coronary arteries were reported to be very large and the walls of the vessels showed a minimal amount of atherosclerosis. Nevertheless, the fatty deposits were there. Whether the large coronary arteries enabled him to develop the superb heart and circulatory system needed by a champion athlete, or whether the years of exercise training developed his large blood vessels, is a matter of speculation. Even though there was some coronary atherosclerosis, the large size of the arteries prevented any restriction of blood flow to the heart muscle.

The remarkable feature of De Mar's case was the demonstration that an American male, well past sixty years of age could continue to be in tip-top physical condition. It should be noted, however, that even De Mar's level of physical activity did not prevent atherosclerotic deposits. If indeed it could be proved that De Mar's coronary circulation and heart could have been developed solely by exercise by showing similar developments in other individuals, it would be a significant contribution to the knowledge of the use of exercise in preventing heart disease. Unfortunately, such observations are not available.

There is always a great danger in drawing conclusions from "one case" reports. The fallacy of drawing overenthusiastic conclusions from the observations made on the case of De Mar is indicated by the case of one of my former patients when he was approximately forty years old. He was a physiologist who had been a college athlete record-holder and had continued to maintain high levels of physical activity, carefully controlling his body weight. By the time he reached fifty years of age he was still exercising vigorously running as much as six miles a day. His endurance runs at a relatively fast jog were interspersed with short bursts of top speed. From what has been said thus far about exercise and the work of the heart, it is clear that such rapid bursts of speed increase the work of the heart enormously for short periods of time.

During one morning exercise period, his running mate noted that he was no longer with him. They had paused for a short time to rest along the roadside and then had resumed running. The running partner turned back to see what had happened to him and found him lying at the side of the road. He had apparently collapsed as soon as he resumed running and died instantaneously. An examination of the heart showed extensive atherosclerosis of all major coronary arteries, even though the heart muscle presented the features of an athletic heart: the muscle appeared strong, and the ventricular cavities of adequate dimensions. This observation is important since it demonstrates the ability to develop a strong vigorous heart muscle even in the face of advanced coronary disease. Careful examination of the heart muscle showed an area of infarction, or acutely damaged heart muscle.

This individual, who regularly engaged in a high level of vigorous exercise and maintained the capacity of an endurance athlete, had extensive coronary artery disease and died during exercise from an acute heart attack. It is pertinent to question whether this man would have died if he had used a somewhat less ambitious exercise program, particularly avoiding peak exertion. He might have maintained an adequate heart muscle for his daily requirements without imposing peak overloads that could precipitate an acute heart attack.

Occasionally accidents provide an opportunity to note the presence and degree of coronary artery disease in relatively young fit individuals, such as a young Air Force pilot who proved to have coronary atherosclerosis. When I first saw him, he was in peak physical condition. He had been a distance runner and had regularly engaged in physical activities from his early days at West Point (when he nearly made the Olympic Team) to the time of his accidental death. He was relatively tall and lean, with no evidence of significant body fat deposits upon physical examination. He, like the physiologist, enjoyed the "well-balanced American diet," with liberal quantities of dairy products, including eggs and milk. An unfortunate accident claimed his life when he was only in his mid-thirties, and the autopsy revealed extensive atherosclerosis of his coronary arteries, with almost complete obliteration of at least one major artery and extensive obstruction of a second branch. Basically, he had only one major artery appreciably free of disease to provide blood supply to the heart muscle.

This man had been studied very carefully. During maximum-exercise testing on the treadmill, he turned in scores compatible with endurance athletes training for the Olympics. He commonly demonstrated a resting heart rate in the low forties. By all standards he had the appearance on medical examination of an endurance athlete. He was able to develop a heart of an athlete with this capability despite the obviously long-standing, extensive coronary artery disease. This case, like the preceding one, demonstrates the ability to develop a strong and capable heart muscle, even in the presence of coronary atherosclerosis. This is good evidence that nature's redundant system for supplying blood to the heart muscle, is adequate enough to enable one to develop a reasonably strong heart. This is a strong argument against the concept that in many people the coronary blood flow to the heart muscle is the limiting factor to exercise.

Still another case was brought to my attention when a famous pilot was killed in an aircraft accident. He was an exercise enthusiast and had encouraged his fellow pilots to pursue a similar course. Although he was over forty years of age at the time of his death, an examination of his heart showed very large coronary arteries with minimal or no significant evidence of atherosclerotic deposits. As in the case of De Mar, one might conclude that exercise had protected his coronary arteries. The four cases are interesting—two showing minimal disease, one showing disease with an acute heart attack precipitated during exercise, and the other showing extensive disease with no known episode of a heart attack. Clearly, vigorous, regular physical activity is not a panacea; it does not prevent coronary artery disease, and by the same token coronary artery disease may not prevent exercise.

Exercise Can Kill You

Russian scientists have demonstrated that in rabbits exercise in the presence of extensive coronary artery disease can cause damage of the heart muscle, like that resulting from acute heart attacks. The amount of muscle damage produced is directly related to the amount of exercise imposed upon the diseased animals. Exercise may be damaging to the heart when it significantly exceeds one's regular level of activity. A crash exercise program or the exercise testing of individuals who are not accustomed to regular exercise may cause a heart attack. Several examples of such attacks have occurred when the Royal Canadian Air Force 5 BX procedure was used as a testing device. The 5 BX program was not originally designed or recommended for this purpose. The problem is exemplified by one individual who reported to a facility for testing his exercise capacity, as scored by the 5 BX system. He had not been exercising regularly and had not been trained to what was considered an optimal level for an individual of his age. During the testing, he collapsed and developed a fatal irregularity of his heart —ventricular fibrillation.

Many a well-intentioned exercise program to improve the general health and physical fitness has come to an abrupt end by the improper use of exercise. A military commander may decide that it is time to get all of his troops "in shape," and then orders all hands to fall out for an hour of vigorous exercise. Sometimes the middle-aged, overweight, unfit individuals "fall out" permanently, dying with an acute heart attack, causing exercise to be discredited and the program to be discontinued at once. Such events in no way discredit the use of exercise in prevention of heart disease. They merely discredit the uninformed use of exercise by the naïve enthusiast.

A good many of the young men with acute heart attacks during World War II dropped dead suddenly during physical activity. Subsequent study of their coronary arteries often demonstrated occlusion or clotting of a coronary artery prior to the time of exercise and death. These findings suggested that the blood supply to part of the heart muscle had already been compromised by a preceding blockage. The heart muscle might have survived the arterial block-age, had no unusual demands been placed upon it, but exercise at a critical time can exceed the auxiliary blood supply to the heart muscle and cause muscle damage, irregularity, and death.

The cases of an Air Force cadet and an Air Force officer always remind me of the danger of drinking cold fluids immediately after exercise. One was only twenty years old and the other was twenty-four. On different occasions, each had been playing football. Neither had any features that would suggest he should be susceptible to a heart attack. Both were vigorous young men, with normal blood-fat studies, and neither was overweight. After a vigorous football game, the younger man had downed a very cold soft drink; the other drank large amounts of ice-cold water. Shortly after drinking cold fluids, both began to experience chest pain and developed an acute heart attack. Why or how drinking cold fluids precipitates an acute heart attack is a mystery. As the heart rests directly on the diaphragm over the stomach, the heart muscle can be chilled and the electrocardiogram changed by drinking cold fluids. Cold apparently may precipitate coronary artery spasm and occlude the blood supply to the heart muscle. Regardless of the validity or reason for incriminating cold fluids, it is a wise precaution not to drink cold fluids after severe exertion until after resting at least fifteen minutes.

There are numerous examples of ill-advised exercising and exercise testing in individuals who have been inactive and even in persons who have just gotten up after prolonged bed rest. The rule of thumb to follow to avoid being killed by exercise is to increase gradually the amount of exercise above your daily level. Do not expect to accomplish miracles in a single exercise period; give your heart muscle a chance to develop enough strength and the coronary arteries a chance to develop enough capacity to insure that you are not overworking your heart or coronary circulation.

You Can Exercise Even If You Have Heart Disease

Obviously, considering the extent of coronary artery disease in the United States and other industrialized nations, and the large number of individuals who do engage in different levels of physical activity at various intervals, the presence of heart disease does not prevent one from exercising. The two cases of athletic individuals who had extensive coronary artery disease, yet exercised regularly, demonstrate that even when obstruction to the blood flow to the heart muscle exists, relatively high levels of exercise can be carried out. The heart tends to compensate for or adjust to the different defects it may have. As long as these compensatory mechanisms are satisfactory, there is little evidence of heart disease. Some individuals with certain valvular defects of the heart can exercise without significant limitation. Some have held athletic records and engaged in regular competition.

While examining United States Air Force pilots, I saw a number of individuals with disease of the aortic valve who had no significant limitation despite their defect. Several of these persons could exercise on the treadmill at levels comparable to the endurance athletes training for the Olympics. These individuals would never have known they had any difficulty with their heart had it not been discovered on an annual examination. These observations emphasize that one need not become a cardiac invalid unless he has severe or extensive heart disease. The vast number of individuals with minor valvular defects of the heart, or the much greater number of individuals with silent coronary artery disease, can and should lead a normal life, including adequate amounts of physical activity.

There are, of course, specific times when physical activity should be avoided. One of these times is immediately after an acute heart attack. Unless there is a specific and well-defined reason for not living a normal, physically active life, all individuals should have some program of regular exercise, even if this is limited to a daily walk. One has to have relatively severe heart disease or have sustained a very recent heart attack for a moderate walk on level terrain to pose any significant threat to the heart and circulation.

You're Not Too Old to Exercise

Many individuals think that once you're past forty years of age you are too old to exercise. Nothing can be further from the truth. As pointed out earlier, many of the ritual dancers in African tribes are over seventy years of age. These vigorous individuals exercise regularly without difficulty. Many an older person plays a great deal of tennis regularly with no significant impairment to the function of the heart. True, most of these individuals do not have the same level of physical stamina they had when they were twenty years old, but there are many of these vigorous older people who have better cardiovascular function with a better endurance heart muscle than many soft twenty-year-old overfed and underfit youths.

Considering the combined effects of high altitude and exercise, it is interesting that in 1963 the Bulgarian Olympic Committee's *Bulletin d'Information* reported that a group of Bulgarians with an average age of sixty-three, and an age span of fifty-five to eighty, hiked in the mountains at altitudes between 4900 and 8900 feet. The hike lasted for thirty days and covered 435 miles. All members of the group remained in good health throughout the hike. It is not age that determines whether or not you can exercise. The important factor is *how* you exercise.

Why Athletes Die of Heart Disease

The exercise antagonists frequently try to find examples of someone who has been harmed by exercise. Such individuals have the philosophy that if they have the urge to exercise but are patient and wait long enough, the urge will go away. A question often raised in discussions with such persons is why so many individuals who have been prominent in the athletic field die in their middle forties of heart disease. The key to the answer is "have been prominent." If they had not been prominent their deaths would not have warranted any major news coverage and might have gone unnoticed, along with the other hundreds of thousands of Americans who die every year from heart disease.

Another important point is that most of them "have been" athletes. A prominent college football star may be an All-American athlete when he is twenty-five, but after football days his habit pattern changes completely. He may become president of the local bank, or he might be prominent in the Chamber of Commerce. It is a safe bet that he will have moved from the football field to the office. With this transition, his level of physical activity decreases and his requirement for calories is much smaller. A college football player may utilize well in excess of five thousand calories a day without gaining weight. As an office worker he may need only 2500 calories a day. Unless our "former athlete" cuts down on his food he will load down his body with excess calories. In a short time his once strong and firm muscles become soft and flabby, and what was once protein is replaced by fat. The extra calories are stored as fat deposits around the body. In a few years, what was once a superb athlete becomes a middle-aged, fat, flabby man. It is not an athlete who died of heart disease—it is a former athlete, who like many other victims of heart disease, has become the fat and unfit prey of the great killer.

Aside from the former athletes who succumb to heart disease, a few young individuals including adolescents and school children die suddenly from exercise. These are relatively uncommon deaths and many of them are caused by abnormal blood supply to the heart muscle. Occasionally an individual will be born with only one major coronary artery (either the right or left) as opposed to the usual two vessels, or with some other abnormality that prevents part of the heart muscle from getting enough blood. When such an individual engages in acute severe physical activity, this defect may suddenly compromise his heart, causing him to have an acute heart attack. In other instances, there may be abnormalities from birth in the blood supply to the vital pacemakers of the heart. This can cause major irregularities of the heart in young people, or the heart may actually stop. These rare instances, commonly associated with birth defects of the heart, are not a justifiable argument against the appropriate use of exercise to help thwart the great killer.

Watch Out for the Mountains

As long as one does not engage in significant levels of physical activity, traveling from sea level to most of the mountainous routes involving land travel is not likely to impose any significant additional load upon the heart and circulation unless such an individual has advanced disease. At altitudes in excess of five thousand feet, one should begin to pay more attention to the combined effects of exercise and altitude. The oxygen pressure in the air sacs of the lungs decreases and the oxygen content in the circulating blood is less. This increases the amount of blood flow needed by the heart muscle. The effects of exercise and high altitude are additive. Exposure to moderately high altitude may be safe and a given level of exercise at sea level alone may not be harmful, but the combination of exercise and hypoxia can exceed the capacity of a compromised circulation.

An individual in peak physical condition tolerates these combined stresses better than the individual who is less fit. A wise thing to do upon initial exposure to high altitude is to limit your physical activity below the customary amount at sea level; even walking may prove to be more exertion than expected. After a few days, the exercise level may be gradually increased; but *you should avoid reaching your usual level of physical exertion* until two weeks have passed. This two-week period is necessary for the bone marrow to produce an adequate amount of additional red blood cells. These additional cells enable more oxygen to be carried per unit of blood. The blood going to the heart muscle then will be able to carry more oxygen. This will enable the heart to function more as it did at sea level and will sharply decrease the additional demands that altitude has made for the blood flow to the heart muscle. At this point, the amount of exercise can gradually be increased to the customary amount at sea level.

Many individuals are unaware of the combined effects of altitude and exercise. Vacationers living at sea level go to mountainous areas and immediately proceed to hike, fish, and golf, far surpassing the amount of their daily activities at sea level. The result is not unlike what happened to the exercised, atherosclerotic rabbits in the Russian experiments mentioned on page 147. Many a hunter, leaving his office and going to the mountainous areas, is an easy victim for the great killer. If you are planning a trip to the mountains you can take some precautionary measures in advance. These include weight reduction (if you are moderately overweight) and an effort to improve your level of physical activity. These two factors will enable you to enjoy your vacation in the mountains with a significantly decreased risk to your health and life.

Should You Exercise after a Heart Attack?

Immediately after a heart attack, the major problem is to develop sufficient blood supply to the remaining areas of living heart muscle. This process is slow. Just as it takes time to grow a vine, it takes time to grow and develop new blood vessels. The heart muscle normally supplied by the freshly occluded coronary artery desperately needs all of the blood it can get, even if one is resting. Not overloading the heart muscle will give the injured area a chance to heal better and form a firmer, smaller scar.

After a period of three or four weeks, depending upon how the individual has done after the acute attack, a gradual increase in physical activity may be beneficial, but the level of activity at this point means walking about the room enough to take care of one's personal hygiene. Gradually the amount of walking and physical activity may be increased. The pace of the increased physical activity has to be determined on an individual basis, but it should never be so rapid nor the exercise so severe as to compromise the remaining blood supply to additional areas of heart muscle. Well after the attack has occurred, progressively longer periods of simple walking is the best program. Exercise activity beyond and above this level of exercise within the weeks immediately following an acute heart attack, is not advisable. Although walking may gradually be increased, usually within six weeks of the occurrence of an acute heart attack, nothing more than moderate walks is advisable until a period of three months has passed.

When people exercise at an earlier date, it often represents an unnecessary and ill-advised risk. A little patience and a gradual increase in exercise can go a long way toward saving enough of the heart muscle, and developing sufficient blood supply for it, to insure the capacity for normal physical activity in pursuit of life's pleasures after adequate recovery. Pushing an exercise program too soon can result in additional muscle damage and a lower limit of the capacity of the heart and circulation as a final result. For optimal recovery and maintenance of optimal capacity of the heart and circulation, the gradual approach is the wise approach. Gradualism, however, must not be extended into undue procrastination or failure to return to adequate levels of physical activity. An individual who has survived a heart attack and regained reasonable function of his heart does much better and lives longer if he resumes an appropriate level of daily activity.

How to Test Yourself for Fitness

The first step on deciding whether or not you are really fit is to look at yourself in the mirror. There are very few fat individuals who are really optimally fit. If there is an appreciable quantity of excess fat about your waist, around your back, or in the buttocks, you are not at an optimal level of fitness. One can carry a certain amount of fat and still be reasonably fit; but these individuals are exceptions. The fatty tissue acts as a pack or weight would on a racehorse. It increases the work of the heart when an individual is accomplishing any task that involves his body weight. One should not take comfort in being fat and still maintaining a relatively high degree of fitness, because the presence of excess fat deposits probably means fat deposits in the coronary arteries and possibly in the arteries to other vital organs.

One of the simplest tests for judging your level of fitness is taking your heart rate while lying down. In women, a resting heart rate below seventy-five beats per minute is a reasonable value. In men in good physical condition, the resting heart rate should be less than seventy beats per minute. If it is faster you must consider the possibility either that your daily exercise program is not adequate or that the effects of tobacco, coffee, and alcohol may be the causative factors. If your resting heart rate is approaching ninety beats per minute and you are not anxious, then something is wrong. Frequently this something is flabbiness or the excess use of tobacco, coffee, or alcohol. Remember, well-trained athletes frequently have resting heart rates below fifty beats per minute, as do other individuals in optimum levels of fitness.

A second useful test is to observe what happens to your heart rate while standing motionless. If your heart rate rises over fifteen beats per minute with standing or exceeds one hundred beats per minute while standing, you are not in optimal condition. The test is best performed by standing quietly for two or three minutes. The heart rates of well-trained individuals in good health and not suffering from anxiety frequently will increase less than ten beats per minute.

There is a surprisingly large number of American men whose heart rates approach or even exceed one hundred beats per minute in their normal afternoon activities. These frequently noted high heart rates are directly related to a lack of physical activity, the use of large amounts of tobacco during conferences and interviews, and finally the ever-present office coffeepot. These factors are probably much more significant in producing unphysiologically high heart rates than the stress and excitement of the day's activities.

A third way of checking your level of fitness, providing you haven't already flunked the first two procedures, is to do some mild exercise for approximately a minute, such as running in place at a modest jog; then lie down and check your heart rate immediately after stopping exercise. If your heart rate is a hundred beats per minute or more you could significantly improve your health status. The sooner your heart rate returns to a resting level, and provided that resting level is well below a hundred beats per minute, the more likely that you are in optimal physical condition. The longer the heart rate stays high after mild exercise, the greater the probability that you are unfit or need to change your way of living.

Occasionally an exercise enthusiast advises individuals to undergo testing procedures involving extensive exercise. Just as the misuse of the Royal Canadian Air Force 5 BX procedure for testing can cause death, so can any other ill-advised testing procedure. Most of these recommendations are not made by heart specialists, although they are sometimes recommended by physicians who should know better. There are diet quacks, but there are also exercise quacks. If you want good advice concerning heart disease and exercise, it is well to get your advice from a heart specialist. It is a sound principle in accepting advice—written or verbal—to know its source. Many books and pamphlets on exercise contain recommendations that are worse than useless—they are dangerous. Do not allow anyone to talk you into running as far as you can go. If you undergo maximum exercise testing be sure it is recommended by a heart specialist— not an athletic coach or a physician who has become an exercise enthusiast and is inexperienced in heart disease problems.

How to Start an Exercise Program

The first question is whether you really should begin an exercise program. Certainly, if you have recently had a heart attack, unless your doctor has advised some form of physical activity, you should not begin such a program on your own. Individuals who knowingly have some form of heart disease, such as rheumatic heart disease or a congenital heart defect, should not try to engage in endurance athletics without their doctor's advice. There is a practical difference between the level of physical activity required for normal enjoyment of average living as opposed to trying to set new athletic records. If you are one of the very large number of individuals who has not had a recent heart attack or had heart disease diagnosed by your doctor, and want to insure yourself of the advantages that can be achieved by exercise, then you can and should begin such a program. You could begin a gradual exercise program if you have had a heart attack a number of months ago and have progressed adequately without recurrence of chest pain or other major difficulties. At the beginning you should limit the amount you might hope to achieve. Young individuals, if they have the time and inclination, should really strive to build gradually to a level of peak physical conditioning.

All overweight individuals should start reducing before beginning any form of vigorous exercise. Weight reduction will immediately reduce the workload imposed on your heart by physical activity. If you are overweight the only addition you should make to your regular level of physical activity is simple walking, until significant weight reduction has been accomplished. It is dangerous for the middle-aged overweight American man to start a *vigorous* exercise program without first losing weight. After long periods of inactivity your body must make many adjustments before you can safely do vigorous exercise, particularly if the exercise involves running, jogging, or other activity involved in supporting the body weight. The tendons in the ankles and knees need to be strengthened; the tone and tension in the leg muscles need to be improved. Walking and starting at a low level of exercise with a very gradual increase in activity helps to prevent soreness in the legs produced by the increased jars and shocks to the joints and muscles.

The best way for an individual who has not been pursuing a regular exercise program to get started is to walk, walk, walk. At first, a fifteen-minute walk a day might be sufficient. After four or five days, the duration of the walk should gradually be increased, being careful not to overdo it at any one time. The gradual increase in walking time should continue until you can walk an hour or an hour and a half continuously, without undue fatigue. It may require three to four weeks for an individual who is not in very good shape to develop enough tolerance to walk this long. Walking exercises should continue for a period of at least a month before trying to add any other form of exercise. It is possible, if you are young, reasonably vigorous, and not too badly out of shape, to accelerate this program. You may initially be able to walk an hour without undue fatigue. If this is true you should keep it up for a couple of weeks and then begin a more vigorous exercise program.

Perhaps the most effective forms of exercise for training the heart and generally improving the circulation are those that involve walking, running, jogging, or endurance-type activities. These are all forms of activity that can be carried out at a reasonably low level for an extended length of time. There are many different concepts as to how a person might gradually improve his exercise capacity. If you have an opportunity to do your exercise in a gymnasium or outdoors, the walking program can be extended gradually by jogging fifty steps then walking five minutes and jogging another fifty steps, then walking another five minutes. Over a long period of time the jogging can gradually be increased so that it is possible for you to jog at a very slow comfortable pace for thirty minutes to an hour.

Another approach to the problem, particularly if you must do your exercise indoors, is to run in place. If one does stationary running, particular care must be taken in the way the running is done. The heel should be allowed to sink to the floor gently with each step, thereby minimizing the shock to the ankle, its tendon, and the calf muscle. The first four days you should run only one hundred steps, counting one step each time the left foot hits the floor. The rate of running should be between seventy-five and a hundred steps a minute. After four days of exercising at that level, unless you have calf or leg soreness, you can increase the level of exercise by fifty steps to 150 steps in one and one-half minutes. If there is any soreness in the ankles or the calf you should continue at the level of one hundred steps a day until all of the soreness has disappeared. After four days at each level of exercise, you can increase the amount of exercise by fifty steps, still maintaining the same rate of seventy-five to one hundred steps a minute. This provides a gradual increase in the level of activity. Any time soreness occurs you should drop back to the previous step level and stay there until the soreness has disappeared.

Under no circumstances should the rate of progression increase any more rapidly than fifty steps every four days. Gradually, at this rate, you will achieve a level of 1500 steps in fifteen to twenty minutes. This level of exercise is adequate to do a great deal toward burning excess calories and improving the general state of the heart and circulation. Usually, the exercise will become easier once you have passed the five hundred-step or five-minute level. The important purpose of the exercise is not to run as fast as you can or as long as you can but to do it regularly seven days a week for fifteen minutes at a rate of one hundred steps a minute. Almost everyone can afford to use fifteen minutes a day to help maintain the function of his heart and circulation. You can carry out this form of exercise wherever you are—in your own home or in a distant hotel, during rain or shine, during heat or blizzard.

There is no reason why you can't run back and forth indoors if you have enough space to move around instead of standing exactly in one spot. The movement back and forth will help to relieve the monotony. Exercising with the aid of music is beneficial and some people find this pleasant, somewhat like dancing.

Another way to counteract boredom is to watch television while running in place. There is no reason that the newscast can't be watched during such activity. There isn't any law that requires a person to sit in an overstuffed chair in front of a television set with his eyes glued to the screen, a martini in one hand, potato chips and cheese dip in the other. If you want to be well informed, you might develop your exercise period parallel with a time to watch the news. This way you can get your exercise and know what's going on in the world at the same time.

Although it has some disadvantages in terms of portability, particularly for the busy executive who must travel from one location to another, a stationary bicycle in the home is a convenient exercise tool. It removes some of the jarring stress on the legs and ankles that is associated with running. If you elect to use a bicycle which has a variable load setting, set it at a load which is comfortable for you and pedal at a regular moderate speed that doesn't tire or overtax you. Try this for a minute a day for the first four days then gradually increase the amount an additional minute every five days until you can exercise at a reasonable load for a period of fifteen minutes. If your heart rate increases too much or if you experience any evidence of discomfort with any form of exercise, you should stop immediately and lie down.

Once you have achieved the capacity to run in place fifteen minutes a day, or walk and intermittently jog an hour a day, and wish to add additional exercises, you may do so provided that at no time the level is increased too rapidly. You can start doing sit-ups and push-ups a few at a time, then gradually increase their number. These additional exercises will help strengthen your other muscles as well as improve your posture and physical well-being. They will also enable you to extend your exercise period, thereby utilizing more calories. A mild calisthenic period built up to occupy a period of from fifteen to thirty minutes a day, carried out on a regular basis, will go a long way toward providing an adequate exercise program for almost anybody. It may not train you to compete in the Olympics but it might prevent you from having a heart attack or enable you to survive one if you do.

A frequent complaint about developing an exercise program is that it takes too much time. Obviously, fifteen minutes a day is not a great time requirement. It is interesting that a large number of the individuals who offer this excuse are the same ones who have two to three hours a day to spend for eating and drinking—their overweight bodies show the results. These individuals could profitably take less time to eat less calories and use this additional time period to develop an exercise program.

A number of people feel that when they come home from a day in the office they are simply too tired to exercise. This sensation of fatigue is often related to a lack of exercise. If they have the will-power to do a modest amount of exercise, to take even a short walk, the physical activity will help to energize them and overcome their fatigue.

A popular misconception is that you can substitute one form of exercise for another. You can't. Different muscles are used for different activities. I know an All-American swimmer who, after engaging in distance running, had sore and painful ankles to the extent of being unable to walk. Never engage strenuously in any unaccustomed activity. If you haven't played tennis for six months, develop your skill gradually, not all in one afternoon. Gradual development of any form of exercise is the key to success without danger or discomfort.

Rewards for Fitness

Several benefits can be expected from a successful exercise program. There is an improvement in the blood flow to your heart muscle. The development of additional blood supply and the development of connections between the different arteries significantly improves the likelihood that an occlusion of any one vessel will not produce major damage to your heart muscle. It can't provide a guarantee but it will improve your chances. In this sense, it serves as an insurance policy. There are a number of studies which suggest that sedentary people have a much higher incidence of heart attacks than active people. Medical studies in Israel demonstrated that white-collar workers had at least four times as many heart attacks as laborers. Comparison of bus drivers to standing conductors and of mail carriers to postal clerks also suggest that the more active occupations are associated with a lower incidence of heart attacks. When individuals are admitted to a hospital with a heart attack, the patients who previously had followed a satisfactory exercise program have a better chance of survival than those who had been relatively sedentary.

While adequate exercise clearly has many advantages, it should not be used as "an excuse to eat." There is a strong tendency in individuals who like to eat, to consider that a minimal amount of exercise provides an immunity against the need to control diet and eliminate excess ingestion of fat and calories. Eventually, these individuals pay for their fantasy. The answer to the question of exercise and diet is very simple. If you are fat—reduce. If you are flabby—exercise.

Children and Exercise Habits

The best time to influence development of the human body is during growing years, since stronger and better muscles, including the heart muscle, can be developed during this period. This, of course, does not exclude the fact that mature and older individuals can make significant improvements, but for optimal capacity the best opportunity is to begin such training during childhood. Children should be encouraged to be physically active. The activity stimulates the growth of their heart muscle and its strength and an adequate blood supply for it. Active children approach adult life with a very good blood supply to the heart muscle. Increased interest in athletics and early training may well be a factor in the achievement eventually of new athletic records on an annual basis.

The wise course is to start your child on an exercise program early in life; let him enjoy the advantages of running, swimming, and the sports of his choice. He should be encouraged to take pride in his level of physical fitness and his performance ability. Too often parents become enamored with such team sports as Little League baseball, basketball, or football. Team sports are wonderful for paternalistic pride, but very few adults play football or basketball. It is a lot easier to be able to continue playing tennis and to find one person to play it with, once the school years are over, than it is to find enough people to play football. A wise parent and a wise athletic director, who are truly interested in developing in children the exercise habits which can be used for a lifetime, will encourage the development of skills in tennis, handball, squash, swimming, skiing, and other athletics that don't require large teams. If a child learns to do these well and enjoys them, the probabilities are that he will continue to be physically active to an adequate degree throughout his life-span. Attention to these types of sports versus the team efforts could well start your child on a program which could prevent him from becoming a victim of heart disease.

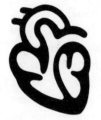

CHAPTER VIII

Man Does Not Die from Fat Alone

WHAT A PERSON EATS is only one factor in the development of heart disease. There is a strong suspicion that if one was clever enough to choose his parents properly, he may have an inherited immunity to heart disease. What effect, if any, does tobacco have upon the development of heart disease? Is it really true that alcohol is good for the heart? Should you drink coffee or tea? Is man's ambitious and aggressive nature his real enemy? These and a host of other factors are part of the sociological and cultural patterns that may influence heart disease.

Red Man's Revenge

When the European came to the western hemisphere, not only did he find potatoes, corn, and the turkey, but the American Indian introduced him to tobacco. Until then, western civilization had never known the joys of tobacco-stained teeth, of breath and clothing impregnated with the odor of nicotine. The prudent American Indian restricted the use of his tobacco leaf to the ceremonial smoking of pipes. A social gathering occasioned by the meeting of two chiefs, or strangers meeting in harmony, was the reason for pipe smoking; thus, even in the culture of the American Indian, tobacco had social status. It did not take the white man long to adopt the Indian ceremonial leaf and chew it, snuff it, roll it in little white papers for smoking, use it as a twisted tobacco leaf similar to the modern cigar, or puff on an innumerable variety of pipes.

Long after the last small groups of American Indians were herded to the reservation, the spirit of the peace pipe smoked in a thousand broken promises remained to reap its revenge. Tobacco and its consequences became a worldwide part of living. Cigarette consumption grew and grew until in the United States and other western industrialized nations, the man who didn't smoke was an exception. Not to be outdone, women gradually but somewhat later took up the habit with increasing frequency, until today smoking among women is commonplace. A few decades ago, a young mother with a baby in her arms and a cigarette dangling from her mouth would have been cause for local gossip—today it is the expected. There was a time when a high school student caught smoking was expelled. Now the problem is how to prevent grade school children from acquiring an early cigarette habit. The increasing mountain of evidence of the adverse effect of cigarette smoking has been associated with a decrease in smoking in certain selected segments of the population—notably physicians. These isolated examples of reduced smoking in knowledgeable groups has had little impact upon the total consumption of tobacco.

As early as 1908, the medical profession learned that tobacco could cause gradual obliteration of the lumen of the arteries (*Berger's disease*). Patients with this problem in the arteries of the legs noted severe pain and cramping of the leg muscles upon walking. The pain was usually relieved when the exercise was terminated or after a period of motionless standing. Individuals who persisted in smoking after these difficulties were noted usually developed gangrene of part of their limbs and had to have amputations. The inveterate nature of the cigarette smoker exemplified itself even during these early observations of tobacco's adverse effect upon health. A particularly habituated individual, after having both legs and one hand amputated, would still be smoking a cigarette on his way to the operating room to lose the remaining hand. Regression of the disease was noted in many instances when smoking was completely and permanently stopped. These observations led to early study of the influence of tobacco on the blood vessels to the peripheral parts of the body, namely the skin, hands, and feet. It was soon determined that nicotine caused a spasm or severe contraction of the terminal arteries.

After intermittent chest pain from heart disease was observed, occasionally individuals were found in whom smoking was a precipitating factor. While these cases were not numerous, they were relatively specific and soon came to be labeled as *tobacco angina*. Why some individuals were afflicted in this way and others were not remained a mystery. It seemed that certain individuals were particularly sensitive to tobacco, just as some individuals have an allergic reaction to ragweed pollen while others do not.

It remained for the advent of epidemiological studies within the past two decades to really raise a red alert on the role of cigarette smoking in health. Not only was cigarette smoking implicated in the rapid increase in the dreaded cancer of the lung, but its association with an increased frequency of heart attacks was clearly established. In this connection it is important to emphasize that the association between cigarette smoking and heart disease has not been established as a cause and effect relationship, that is, proof that tobacco causes heart disease. What has been established on a statistical basis is that individuals who smoke a great deal, as a group, are the individuals who are far more likely to have heart attacks. Whether this increased likelihood is due to tobacco itself or to some other socio-cultural factor related to smoking in coronary artery disease, cannot now be stated. The fact that there is a relationship between cigarette smoking and heart disease, however, is sufficiently well established that *there is only one chance in one hundred that such a relationship could exist as a pure coincidence.* In men, who are high-risk candidates for heart attacks anyway, heavy smoking may be associated with a threefold increase in the frequency of heart attacks. Recently Dr. David Spain of New York reported that heavy smoking in men with coronary-artery disease was associated with. sudden death at a younger age. Individuals who smoked twenty or more cigarettes daily died sixteen years sooner on the average than nonsmokers. At the time of death the average age of nonsmokers was 63.2 years (range of 61 to 69 years), while the average age of the heavy smokers was 47.4 years (range of 35 to 62 years). Women smokers do not escape such an association either. There is a definite increase in the frequency of heart attacks among women smokers as opposed to nonsmokers.

The difference in smoking habits between populations of men

and women may be one of the factors for the disproportionately high incidence of heart attacks in men as opposed to women. As the studies have progressed, the association with heart disease has suggested that the more one smokes, the greater will be the risk of a heart attack. There may be other factors which influence the association. The person who inhales the cigarette smoke deeply, to the bottom of the lungs, and smokes the entire cigarette, is undoubtedly absorbing an appreciably greater amount of nicotine than the person who takes two puffs of the cigarette without inhaling and then extinguishes it in the nearest ashtray. Smoking habits make a great deal of difference in the amount of nicotine and other noxious gases inhaled and absorbed by the body.

Gradually more attention is being paid to factors which may cause an association between the high risk of heart attacks and tobacco which are separate and distinct from the concept that nicotine causes heart disease. A legitimate question can be raised about the differences in the personalities of the smoking population versus the nonsmokers. Is a heavy smoker the tense, driving, ambitious individual? Are heavy smokers generally overindulgers, partaking to excess in other facets, including food and drink? What is the relationship of excessive smoking to an excessive coffee- or tea-drinking habit? Is the level of physical activity for excessive smokers limited to opening one pack of cigarettes after another? These are all legitimate questions which may have some influence on the established association.

In the search for some of the direct effects of nicotine upon the heart and circulation, it has been established that nicotine increases the heart rate. It also increases cardiac output and, at least in a transitory manner, may cause a rise in blood pressure. Because of its constricting action on the terminal arteries, it may diminish the flow of blood to the skin. This will cause a drop in temperature of the fingers and other exposed areas of the skin. There is considerable variation between individuals in the response of their circulatory systems to smoking. Some individuals appear to be hypersensitive with marked changes in blood flow to the skin, while others appear to be less affected.

The role of cigarette smoking in producing the pattern of a deconditioned heart (heart of individuals in poor physical condition) deserves some emphasis. In young healthy pilots, leading relatively active average American lives for individuals of their age group, tobacco is a frequent stimulus to a persistently elevated heart rate. Smokers with resting heart rates approaching ninety beats per minute or more often have a drop in heart rate after stopping the cigarette habit to approximately sixty beats per minute. The direct influence of smoking on the heart rate can be established in many individuals by careful experiments. Shortly after tobacco is eliminated entirely, significant slowing of the resting heart rate can be observed. Upon resuming the habit, soon a marked increase in resting heart rate is again apparent. A cause for unexplained persistent rapid heart rate in otherwise healthy individuals is often cigarettes.

Considering the function of the heart, it is clear that this change is not an economical one. The persistent increased resting heart rate of the smoker helps perpetuate a small heart capable of pumping only a restricted stroke volume. Chronic smoking limits the heart in developing a large stroke volume capacity and the characteristics of an endurance muscle. This may well be a significant factor in the occurrence of heart attacks regardless of what effect nicotine does or does not have upon the coronary arteries to the heart muscle.

Nicotine is a well-established cellular poison. Given in sufficient quantities, it can cause death of nerve or other tissues, just as cyanide or other toxic substances may produce tissue death. It is difficult to imagine that even small amounts of poison utilized on a long-term chronic basis could be beneficial to optimum cellular health. Chronic cigarette smoking is associated with an increased buildup in the blood of carbon monoxide, the same lethal gas emitted in the exhaust fumes of automobiles, produced by incomplete combustion of carbon. This toxin forms a relatively stable bond with the hemoglobin molecules in the red blood cells preventing them from carrying oxygen or carbon dioxide. The accumulation of carbon monoxide in the bloodstream limits the oxygen-transport capacity for each unit of blood. Maintaining a persistent level of carbon monoxide poison throughout the body tissues and the bloodstream, can hardly be considered as beneficial to optimal health or maximum performance.

A number of studies have provided evidence that cigarette smoking is directly related to the depletion of vitamin C from the body. It is well known that vitamin C is a very labile substance, easily destroyed by heat and chemicals. One investigator has stated that smoking one cigarette depletes the body of an amount of vitamin C equivalent to one orange. Clearly, on this basis a twenty-cigarette-a-day smoker would have to consume twenty-one oranges to restore the lost vitamin C. The relationship of vitamin C deficiencies to the development of atherosclerosis has given rise to the question of whether cigarette smoking is a stimulus to atherosclerosis on the basis of depleting vitamin C stores in the walls of the arteries.

Numerous studies have demonstrated that cigarette smoking stimulates release of hormones from the adrenal gland. Some of these hormones are known to have powerful effects upon the heart and circulation, while others are related to the amount of circulating cholesterol and beta-lipoproteins in the bloodstream.

A distinct difference exists between the association of heart disease with cigarette smoking and its relation to cigar or pipe smoking, despite the large amount of nicotine in cigars and in pipe tobacco. One possible explanation is related to the use of the tobacco. A cigar smoker ordinarily does not inhale; even if he does, he is seldom the deep inhaler who draws in the smoke to the bottom of his lungs. The same is true for the pipe smoker who spends more time tamping, packing, and lighting his pipe, puffing and blowing smoke than he does in inhaling the smoke itself. Most pipe smokers do not inhale. Whatever the reason for the association of cigarette smoking to heart disease, these studies definitely suggest that if an individual has such a strong oral urge that he cannot resist sticking something in his mouth, he would be well advised to switch to pipes or cigars, and of these two, pipes are preferable.

Coffee, Tea, or Coke

Drinks that stimulate have become suspect for stimulating more than the mind. Coffee, tea, and the kola nut all contain caffeine. In the age of excess, the waking hours are passed by many with a continuous oral infusion of one or more of these beverages.

Caffeine, like Dexedrine, is a powerful stimulant to the nervous system. While one cup is not likely to create any adverse effect, drinking large amounts can be equivalent to chronic overdosage of "go pills." Just as chronic cigarette smoking can contribute to a persistent elevation of the resting heart rate so can a chronic large intake of coffee, tea, or Coke. In young, healthy, active males, resting heart rates in the middle eighties may decrease more than fifteen beats per minute when these excesses are discontinued. All too frequently patients reporting such symptoms as nervousness, burning of the stomach, or palpitation of the heart receive prescriptions for sedatives or tranquilizers, with no questions asked about the chronic ingestion of nervous stimulants. Often what these individuals need is not another drug but elimination of the one they are already consuming in excess.

An individual who drinks ten or more cups of coffee on a daily basis often experiences withdrawal symptoms—general drowsiness, fatigue, and a persistent headache—if coffee is stopped abruptly. If one elects to quit drinking stimulants, unpleasant reactions of this sort can be avoided by continuing to drink one or two cups of coffee or tea a day for a week, then stopping the habit altogether.

Excessive coffee drinking can cause irregularities of the heartbeat, including palpitation or skipped beats. Stopping the coffee habit may also stop the difficulty. More serious irregularities of the heart have been precipitated even in otherwise healthy individuals. Like prolonged overdosage with Dexedrine and other "no doze" and "go" pills, truly excessive, chronic drinking of stimulants has a significant effect upon the psyche and the total organic system. Individual sensitivity varies, but in general, five cups of coffee or tea a day is excessive. In many individuals, one or two cups a day is not harmful. In sensitive individuals, even one cup of coffee a day can give a nonhabituated person quite a charge, which can be noted by an increase in the heart rate and in general nervousness.

The association of stimulating drinks with coronary atherosclerosis and its complications does not rest on solid ground. Initial enthusiasm for this concept has waned a bit when other factors have been considered. Many individuals who drink large amounts of coffee, tea, and Coke, obviously ingest large amounts of sugar. Some investigators have been able to present a relatively convincing case that the large intake of sugar often used with these beverages, is the main culprit—increasing blood cholesterol and beta-lipoprotein levels and increasing problems of heart disease. While no final answer can be given to this intriguing question now, the well-documented effect of large doses of caffeine and the suspicions concerning the continuous ingestion of large amounts of sugar suggest that the prudent course is to limit one's self to black coffee or unsweetened tea in quantities of less than five cups a day. As in so many other instances, moderation may prove to be the key. Of course, if an individual has evidence of palpitation, a high resting heart rate, or general nervousness, the wise thing to do would be to stop the use of stimulating beverages altogether.

The Drinker's Heart

On occasion, alcohol is properly prescribed in the management of heart disease. This, however, does not suggest that regular alcohol ingestion is beneficial. The idea that alcohol is a noncaloric drink is a complete fantasy. To repeat, each gram of alcohol contains approximately seven calories, exceeded in its caloric value only by fat. It stimulates the appetite or releases inhibition, often resulting in a caloric imbalance with a gain in dangerous fat deposits. Most individuals who are unable to forego alcohol in any quantity are unable to maintain optimal caloric balance or to prevent the accumulation of fat. Dietary measures in such individuals are usually doomed to defeat.

Alcohol finds its best use in heart disease when given in small amounts as a sedative, or for the treatment of the recurrent chest pain angina pectoris. The sedative action of alcohol allays anxiety and prevents its adverse affect on the heart and circulation. Although alcohol has not been demonstrated to increase the blood flow to the heart muscle, in some way, perhaps by decreasing cardiac work and the need of the heart muscle for oxygen, it may relieve or prevent anginal pains.

The chronic alcoholic often has other complications associated with his habit. He is the individual who often drinks and doesn't eat. An impoverished alcoholic, as opposed to the affluent one, is more apt to spend his money for alcohol and have none left for food. Soon these individuals will have vitamin and protein deficiencies which cause abnormalities in the heart muscle and blood vessels. The heart muscle begins to fail, resulting in an accumulation of excessive fluids and death unless the situation is corrected.

Continued use of excessive amounts of alcohol, combined with bad dietary habits, may lead to significant liver damage. Damaged liver cells are no longer able to function in the usual manner, in metabolizing fat and generating cholesterol or beta-lipoproteins. Such persons are in a low risk group as far as heart attacks are concerned. Rather than dying from heart disease they die of liver disease. Trading one illness for another does not appear to be a very satisfactory solution to the problem of atherosclerosis. Some chronic alcoholics consume adequate proteins and vitamins, which seems to protect them from serious liver disease. Chronic alcoholism, without damage to the liver, has no apparent protective effect against atherosclerosis, nor does it appear to decrease the risk of having a heart attack. It does increase the risk of pneumonia and infectious diseases found in those poor souls for whom alcoholism and skid row have become a way of life.

In more recent years, the toxic effect of alcohol on the heart muscle has been clearly established. Ingestion of considerable amounts of alcohol results in direct damage of the heart muscle fibers. Essential cellular enzymes that have leaked out of the cell into the bloodstream are an indication of the damage. Chronic use of alcohol in copious amounts can result in significant heart muscle damage called *alcoholic myocardopathy*. Eventually the damaged heart muscle is no longer capable of functioning efficiently as an endurance muscle and heart failure ensues. The first episode is usually reversible. Stopping alcohol results in complete recovery of the heart. Most of these individuals who have such a problem sooner or later return to the bottle. When alcohol returns, heart disease returns, and with each successive bout the probability of permanent severe heart muscle damage is increased.

Is There a Heart Disease Personality?

The concept that arterial atherosclerosis is aided by gluttony and laziness is a distinct departure from the popular concept that a heart attack had occurred because "poor John was so overworked." Being overfed and underfit is not likely to invoke appropriate sympathetic responses. Some relief to this problem has been afforded by the concept of the heart disease personality. Individuals with different personality patterns were studied in respect to heart disease and circulating blood fats. Investigators identified a personality pattern which they have claimed is associated with higher levels of blood cholesterol and a higher incidence of coronary atherosclerosis with its complications. The personality described was somewhat more flattering and ego-satisfying. The coronary-prone person was found to be a hard-driving achiever, strongly competitive, and seeking recognition with advancement. Such individuals were frequently involved in multiple activities at the same time, meeting numerous deadlines, with a tendency toward a constantly accelerated pace. They had exceptional physical and mental alertness. The propensity for heart attacks in this group far exceeded that for individuals with less ambition or a general "don't give a damn" approach to life. Even individuals who might be classified as "personality slobs" were less inclined to have heart attacks, despite an overlay of persistent anxiety, than the all-American achiever.

It was claimed by the investigators that the differences noted in the personality groupings were independent of cigarette smoking, alcohol ingestion, exercise, and hereditary factors; thus, the observations were related directly to the personality patterns involved. Differences in dietary factors were exonerated, insofar as fat intake was concerned, but there is no evidence that the question of positive or optimal caloric balance with control of dangerous fat deposits, or the question of coffee intake associated with excessive ingestion of concentrated carbohydrates, was considered. While these observations are interesting, they have not gained widespread support. Most scientists feel that the desire and efforts to achieve are in themselves hardly satisfactory explanations for the origin of atherosclerosis. If these personality patterns can be linked to other facets, known to have a more direct association with atherosclerosis, perhaps the problem will be clarified.

In an effort to evaluate the concept that personality factors significantly influence the risk of having a heart attack, Dr. Lawrence Hinkle, Jr., and associates studied 270,000 men employed by the Bell System operating companies. To evaluate the role of personality factors identified as "striving people," "competitive," "restless," and "mobilized," reported by other investigators as primary factors in predisposing to heart attacks, Dr. Hinkle studied people of different occupations, levels of achievement, and education. The study failed to show that men with high levels of responsibility had any greater risk of a heart attack than men with lesser responsibilities. Men with college educations and men successful in realizing their goals actually had a lesser number of heart attacks than less educated or less successful men.

Many prominent individuals with heart disease have been achievers and have continued to achieve in positions requiring great drive and exposure to appreciable stress, long after they have had heart attacks. One need only look at the long list of political figures, headed by former Presidents Eisenhower and Johnson, to be reminded of this fact. There are multitudes of individuals in government, business, and other professions who have similar histories. Ambition and goal-seeking exist among all peoples and are not uniquely associated with those who have a high incidence of heart disease. Even in the most primitive tribes, there is the desire to be the best warrior, the best dancer, the chief, or to compete for the favor of a lady. While the stresses associated with efforts for achievement or goal attainment are no doubt important, there is not sufficient evidence to warrant overemphasis of this factor. It is possible that the effects of drive for achievement and other facets are balanced out in some individuals or peoples by the influence of physical activity or by a significant difference in diet, body-fat control, or other habits.

How Important Is Stress?

The problem in evaluating stress is first defining what is meant by the term, and secondly finding objective ways to measure it. There are numerous types of stress—physical stress from endurance exercise, psychic stress from solving a problem, or stress associated with the anxiety of unavoidable impending danger. It is not likely that the broad variety of different forms of stress can all be equated in the same way. There is a difference between anger and fear of danger. There is a difference between frustration and the stress of running a mile.

Heart rate and blood pressure will rise markedly during periods of stress, for example during difficult aerial maneuvers of high-performance jet aircraft. On the basis of what is known of the work of the heart, clearly this represents increased work by the heart muscle. Such situations may cause heart rates of approximately 150 beats per minute, and there may be a major increase in blood pressure. However, there is a marked variation in the responses of different individuals to this type of stress; in some phlegmatic people the heart rate and blood pressure seem to remain relatively constant, whereas other individuals exhibit a volatile response. Although impending danger is not associated with any increased physical work, the circulatory response is thought to be associated with the outpouring of adrenaline-like substances from the adrenal gland. Chemical substances derived from these secretions are sometimes stored in the heart. Long-term recurrent psychic stress could contribute to changes in heart function. Some investigators have thought that physical activity causes a destruction of these substances stored in the heart muscle, and that the best antidote for mental stress was physical stress. This concept is part of the basis for suggesting that business executives, professional people, jet pilots, and other individuals subjected to stress which cannot be acted out in a physical sense, should have regular physical activity.

Acute stress can and does suddenly raise the blood cholesterol level. This also is thought to be mediated through action of the adrenal gland. In students preparing for final examinations, blood cholesterol levels have been shown to fluctuate wildly within short periods of time. Temporary fluctuations in the blood cholesterol levels of this type have not been proved to be associated with subsequent development of arterial atherosclerosis.

Do Parents Make a Difference?

Individuals with certain inherited metabolic abnormalities, such as diabetes, are more susceptible to atherosclerosis. It has not been proved that atherosclerosis alone is an inherited characteristic. One thing is clear—*having long-lived parents or grandparents is no guarantee against developing atherosclerosis.* Not infrequently individuals whose fathers lived into their eighties and nineties without any particular limitation imposed by their health, find themselves the victim of the great killer in their early fifties. The simple truth is that neither father nor grandfather ate or lived in the same way that the son or grandson does today.

Apparent familiar tendencies, such as heart disease occurring in brothers and sisters, must be regarded with considerable skepticism. The same eating and sociological habit pattern usually engulfs an entire family, making it impossible to isolate those factors which are acquired from those which are inherited. When almost all of the adult male population has a disease, such as atherosclerosis, and when one out of two individuals dies from the complications of this disease, the problem is too widespread to make any separations based on heredity. Individuals who do have a strong family history of disease, however, are well advised to pay particular attention to those measures which decrease the high-risk factors for the complications of the atherosclerotic process. These are the individuals who should eliminate long-standing unfavorable family dietary patterns, eradicate bad personal habits, and maintain appropriate levels of physical activity. Whether the family tendency is inherited or whether it is an acquired socio-cultural pattern, such a program would be advised. The same program, however, ought to be followed by every individual interested in significantly reducing the probability of an early death from heart disease. The possibility of really isolating the question of hereditary factors in heart disease will have to wait for reduction in the high incidence of atherosclerosis. There must be a group of individuals truly free of the disease before any meaningful separation can be made to permit such definite studies.

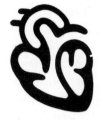

CHAPTER IX

Common Problems and Their Management

THE DISEASES OF MAN change in the course of time. The great plague epidemics are no more. The once dread disease smallpox is almost unknown in the modern, industrialized nations of the world. Each age seems to have its own medical challenge. The circulatory afflictions of man too, have changed. For centuries syphilis was a favorite. The fleshpots of the world teemed with uncontrolled venereal disease. Its toll on the heart and great vessels struck down the young and active. The valves of the heart were destroyed, or growths obstructed the openings of the coronary arteries. In still others, the great aorta stretched and dilated until it ruptured, spilling blood into the chest cavity. Only twenty-five years ago numerous examples of this type of heart disease were available in the hospitals training young doctors, and now such examples are almost nonexistent.

Tuberculosis had its day of glory, affecting the heart and circulation through its effect on the lungs. Even though it has not vanished, its victims are smaller in number. Rheumatic fever, with its crippling effects on youngsters, is preventable and new cases are now uncommon. The grim reaper has been domesticated. Today he sits at your table; he sits with you at your television set; he sits and eats. The mask he wears for his deadly game is the mask of atherosclerosis.

What Is Heart Failure?

Many different diseases can cause heart failure—syphilis, rheumatic fever, diphtheria, thyroid disease, nutritional diseases, high blood pressure, atherosclerosis, and a host of other disorders. The swollen, distended body, filled with excess fluid, has long been a favorite way for heart disease to make its presence known. Heart failure essentially is the failure of the circulation to provide adequate blood flow to the tissues at sufficient pressure to insure normal cell function. At first, the limitation of the circulation may be minimal. Then bit by bit the difference between the capabilities of the circulation and the needs of the tissues increases, producing a vast array of different changes in the body and its function.

One of the first responses the overloaded heart can make is to dilate by lengthening the individual muscle fibers. This improves the mechanical advantage of the heart muscle, much as increasing the length of a lever arm helps to lift a large load. This change in the heart can be seen in X-ray studies.

As the left ventricular muscle loses its ability to pump effectively, the left ventricular cavity continues to enlarge. The muscle fibers eventually become "overstretched," and like an "overstretched" door spring the muscle loses its strength. It is not efficient in ejecting blood, permitting an excess volume of blood to remain in the heart at the end of its contraction. The left atrium has increasing difficulty, and must contract with greater force to expel blood into the over-distended left ventricular cavity. These events result in an increase in pressure within the left ventricular cavity and the left atrium. Eventually, the left atrium dilates as it accumulates an excess volume of blood. The increased pressure in the great left atrial reservoir is transmitted backward into the pulmonary veins returning from the lungs.

Left heart failure causes excess blood to accumulate in the lungs. Blood normally pumped from the right heart to the lungs has difficulty leaving the lungs because of the increased pressure in the left heart. The lungs become congested with blood under increased pressure. The increased pressure in the pulmonary veins prevents fluid from returning to the capillaries in a normal manner. Instead, fluid is pushed out of the circulation and accumulates in the air sacs. The increased amount of watery fluid in the lungs decreases the exchange of gases or limits the normal function of the lungs. They become stiff and lose their elasticity.

Initially, the cardiac output of the failing left heart may be adequate for a person during rest but not during exertion. As an increased amount of blood returns to the right heart with physical activity, the left heart is mechanically incapable of increasing its output. The exercise augments pressure in the pulmonary veins and increases the accumulation of fluid in the lungs. The difficulty in providing oxygen through the wet lungs causes breathlessness. One of the early signs of left heart failure is shortness of breath with exertion. Without successful treatment, the weakening left heart becomes weaker, until even at rest, it is unable to pump adequately—causing persistent shortness of breath.

A large portion of the blood volume is shifted from below the diaphragm into the thorax when one lies down—increasing the amount of blood returning to the right heart. This contributes to the problem of the compromised left heart in pumping blood away from the lungs, and aggravates breathlessness. In severe cases, large amounts of fluid accumulate in the air sacs. This condition is called *pulmonary edema*. The breath sounds are "bubbling" and very noisy. The outlet to the air sacs becomes swollen, creating an obstruction to forcing air out of the inflated lungs. The "wheezing" characteristic associated with the accumulation of fluid in the lungs sounds like an asthmatic attack, which gives rise to the term *cardiac asthma*. When the doctor listens to the wet lungs of a person with left heart failure, he hears the bubbling sounds of excess fluid in the lungs. He may hear the wheezing of cardiac asthma. These sounds are often loud enough to be heart some distance from the patient.

The accumulated fluid in the lungs causes the patient to cough up large amounts of clear, foamy sputum. Clear fluid may accumulate in the space between the lungs and the chest wall in amounts large enough to significantly compress the expandable lungs. The physician often inserts a needle through the chest wall where the fluid has accumulated and simply drains it off. This allows the lungs to expand and improves the lung function. The patient with left heart failure usually finds comfort in sitting upright, decreasing the amount of blood in the thorax by permitting blood to pool below the diaphragm.

In addition to causing excess blood to accumulate in the lungs, the failing left heart does not provide enough blood for the body tissues. This may affect the function of the kidneys. The kidney causes the blood volume to expand by retaining salt and water. The urine output drops precipitously. As long as the right heart is able to accept the increased volume, the amount of blood that accumulates in the lungs increases. A vicious cycle is created; as the total blood volume increases, the blood volume in the lungs increases, further overloading the failing left heart. This in turn further decreases blood flow to the kidney which responds by continuing to increase the blood volume.

While circulatory failure is affecting other organs, the heart undergoes a number of changes. The weakened, overstretched left heart muscle does not contract vigorously, causing the heart sounds to change. The dilated ventricle may cause the valves between the atria and ventricles to fit poorly, allowing a backward leak, which may create a heart murmur. The feeble heart beats at a rapid rate, often with a subnormal stroke volume, creating weak tones and extra sounds, which the heart specialists may call *gallop rhythm*— "the cry of the heart for help."

During left heart failure the patient often sits up, gripping side rails of the bed. The family may be startled one day to see the patient lying flat and breathing comfortably. It resembles a miracle, but things are not always as they seem. The sudden dramatic improvement often signals the failure of the right heart as well. As the blood volume gradually increases in the lungs, the resistance to pumping more blood from the right heart to the lungs gradually increases. When the overworked right ventricular muscle fails, it is no longer able to pump an excessive amount of blood into the lungs. The excessive engorgement of the lungs ceases and blood accumulates behind the right heart. For a time, the lungs may appear to be spared.

The weakened muscle fibers of the right ventricle are stretched to accommodate an increased volume of blood. The pressure increases in the great right atrial reservoir and is transmitted backward along the entire venous system. If the pressure is great enough, the neck veins will begin to stand out, even though the patient is seated upright. Normally, in the upright position, the neck veins are collapsed. The distended neck veins indicate an increase in pressure in the right atrium, capable of supporting a column of blood high enough to reach the head. Each time the right atrium contracts the pulsations in the neck veins can be seen. As the venous pressure increases, the liver, which acts like a gaint sponge extending directly off of large veins joining the vena cava, becomes swollen, enlarged, and tender. This often creates a constant pain in the upper abdomen. The tissues within the liver become swollen and congested with excess fluid. In long-standing cases, areas of scarring and degeneration of liver tissue occurs. In this way heart disease causes liver disease. As the liver becomes diseased, its role in controlling blood sugar, protein metabolism, fat metabolism, and factors related to maintaining the normal clotting mechanism of the blood may all be disturbed.

Increased pressure throughout the venous reservoir of the body prevents the normal return of fluid from the tissues to the circulating blood in the vascular tree. As fluid accumulates in the tissue spaces, swelling of the feet and ankles occurs if the patient is seated upright. Fluid also accumulates in the abdomen. The large liver and excess fluid may cause the abdomen to be markedly distended. This, in turn, limits the movement of the diaphragm and interferes with normal respiration.

Pooling and stagnation of blood can cause blood clots which may dislodge and cause immediate death. The stagnation of blood in the tissues allows the oxygen to be more completely extracted from the hemoglobin in the red blood cells, giving the skin the bluish dusky discoloration of cyanosis.

The increasing blood volume and the progressive weakening of the heart muscle finally result in a recurrence in the accumulation of fluid in the lungs and problems in breathing. The tissues of the body, liver, spleen, intestines, brain, legs, abdominal cavity, lungs, and chest cavities all accumulate excessive amounts of fluid. The poorly oxygenated inadequate blood flow from the heart compromises the blood supply to the heart muscle itself, which further aggravates the condition. Eventually, the patient literally drowns in his own fluids. The entire course of events may be slow or rapid, depending upon the extent of the underlying heart disease.

The picture of advanced heart failure is so typical that most skilled physicians can recognize it on sight. The patient sitting upright, gasping for breath, with distended neck veins and protuberant abdomen, gives immediate evidence of the problem at hand. The remaining question before the physician is the cause of the failure and its treatment. Fortunately, there are a number of things the physician can do in many cases when the heart shows evidence that it is no longer able to meet its demands. Many elderly individuals with advanced heart disease, causing heart failure, have lived for a decade or more after the first evidence of heart failure by using a proper diet and certain medications. Some have enjoyed reasonably active lives well beyond their normal life expectancy.

There Was an Old Lady from Shropshire

Despite all the wonderful recent advances in the management of heart disease, the most important drug is still digitalis—sometimes called a heart stimulant—which was discovered more than two hundred years ago. It is used to correct heart failure and manage certain irregularities of the heart. This valuable medicine was found in a most unusual way by a most unusual English physician, Dr. William Withering, in the latter part of the eighteenth century. One of his favorite hobbies was botany. He had equipped his carriage with a candle, and during his nighttime journeys he often studied botanical works. (Eventually he published a complete book on plants found in England.) In the course of his travels across the English countryside, he learned of the miracles achieved by a brew concocted by an old woman in Shropshire. With his curiosity aroused, he investigated further to find that the old lady would brew tea for patients who had not been benefited by visits to the doctor. Most of the patients helped by the tea had been suffering with so-called dropsy, or heart failure. After drinking the tea over a sufficient period of time, their bodies would be purged of excess fluid, with great loss of water and body weight, their breathing became easier, and their general state of health improved.

As a botanist, Dr. Withering was not long in discovering that the important ingredient of the magic herbal tea was *foxglove*. This observation began the exciting discovery of the most important heart medicine of all time. Withering began experimenting with preparations of foxglove. Soon he learned that he too could benefit a number of patients by carefully adjusting the amount of foxglove given. His studies convinced him of the great value of the foxglove preparation. Despite his outstanding reputation, he spent years attempting to establish the use of the drug in England. His learned colleagues in London and elsewhere decried his observations. With the persistence of a true scientist, he continued to collect evidence and eventually won proper recognition for the use of foxglove in the treatment of heart failure. Until World War II, preparations of foxglove in their original form were commonly used by most heart specialists. These little greenish-colored pills were produced from the dried leaves of the plant. After the essential chemical ingredients of foxglove or digitalis were identified, a large variety of new, purified products was produced. Now there are white pills, and pink pills, indicating different doses of medicine.

The important effects of the family of digitalis medicines that have been developed have remained essentially the same. When used properly they influence the contractility of the muscle fibers in the failing heart. As the strength of the heart muscle fibers is improved, the pumping action is improved—increasing cardiac output. Successful treatment breaks the vicious cycle of heart failure. The excess fluid is poured out, the swelling in the feet and ankles disappears, fluid accumulated in the lungs may vanish, and a swollen and distended abdomen may return to normal size. It is not uncommon for a responsive individual with massive heart failure to lose twenty pounds of fluid. The proper amounts of digitalis may return a heart which has failed to essentially normal function. Such individuals may live many useful years without any significant limitation upon their activities.

Digitalis preparations cannot be used indiscriminately. It is not true that if a little is good, more is better. Excessive amounts of digitalis can have a toxic effect upon the heart muscle, actually causing serious irregularities of the heart or even death. The inclusion of certain digitalis preparations in diet-reducing pills has no justification whatever. Their use by quacks and unscrupulous people for this purpose cannot be condemned too strongly.

Faints

Although ignored for many years by American scientists, the role of breath holding in causing simple fainting was well known in ancient times. In the pre-Christian era, accounts of deaths from breath holding can be found, including one of a captured warrior who was asked about the strength and plans of his band. While appearing to consider his remarks before replying, the warrior covered his face with his hands and bent forward over his knees. Within the grasp of his captors and before them all, he compressed his breath to find an end for himself. There are stories of slaves desiring to end it all who stretched themselves out upon the ground and held their breath until all movement ceased. It was appreciated that young and healthy men, by breath holding, could die suddenly. In a similar way, children holding their breath in fits of anger died. The key to these respiratory maneuvers was simply stopping the heart. If the heart did not beat again, death ensued.

There is a widespread opinion that fainting is an unmanly act— "Only sick people and sissies faint." Fainting suggests the over-wrought female with hysterical swooning episodes. Air Force studies, including flying personnel from the Strategic Air Command, proved that at least forty per cent of the men had experienced one or more episodes of loss of consciousness. With these studies, fainting in young healthy men took on its proper perspective. It was after all a symptom, just as fever is symptom. Almost anyone could faint, the important question was the cause. It might be caused by a needle puncture, an acute illness causing vomiting and diarrhea, an overly sensitive reflex mechanism, or an early sign of our old friend atherosclerosis involving the blood flow to the brain. Studies done in blood banks and the Air Force clearly established one point—the unmanly faint occurred much more frequently in men than in women. Vigorous young athletes, who by all criteria possessed the manly virtues, were as susceptible as any of their associates to fainting in parade formation, immunization-shot lines, and the vast array of human experiences that can precipitate this event.

The hysterical swooning episodes in overwrought females are emotional reactions and not related to the circulation. These are the kind of episodes that occur in bobby-soxers swooning for a matinee idol. The common faint seen in blood banks, parade formations, and other situations is usually associated with a change in the pumping action of the heart or the control of distribution of the cardiac output through changes in the arteries and veins. These changes cause a temporary inadequate blood flow to the brain and fainting. With such episodes, minor convulsive movements or even a major seizure with loss of control of bladder and bowel function can occur. The latter events are uncommon and often associated with brain disease, but they can and do occur with a severe faint.

Simple fainting can occur in normal people following prolonged bed rest, after acute illnesses, and with acute stressful situations of either a physical or emotional nature. Individuals who have recurrent fainting episodes or recurrent dizziness, or who faint for no apparent reason, should seek medical attention. Fainting in the blood bank after giving a pint of blood is one thing, but fainting in the normal course of a day's events, when getting up from the chair or after resting on the sofa, is not a common event.

Occasionally fainting is the only manifestation of a heart attack. In other instances it is an early sign of obstructed blood flow to the brain. Some of these obstructions can be corrected by surgery. Fainting from these causes is more apt to occur in middle-aged or older individuals. Fainting in young individuals prior to physiological maturity, or before age twenty, is not uncommon. Unless it is frequent or spontaneous, it usually has little importance.

In older persons, fainting episodes are sometimes caused by heart block (discussed in Chapter IV). In certain instances a pacemaker or certain medications can be used to insure continued proper action of the heart. In general, unless fainting is caused by a minor injury or occurs in the course of such events as donating blood, you would be wise to seek advice from your physician. If its cause is unimportant, the reassurance is a wonderful tranquilizer, and if it is important it may be possible that something can be done about it.

If someone faints in your presence, the most important thing you can do immediately is to have the person lie down until the acute episode is definitely over. Under no circumstances should he be kept in an upright position. An individual who faints in a phone booth or in a densely packed crowd, preventing him from lying down, may have convulsions or die. If the heart rate has slowed markedly or stopped, lying down often makes it resume beating. When the cardiac output has fallen markedly, lying down helps to insure that a greater portion of blood is pumped to the brain, aiding a prompt recovery.

Coronary Atherosclerosis

The vast majority of adult American men today have coronary atherosclerosis. One of its complications—the acute heart attack—kills approximately a half million people a year. This one complication alone is the leading cause of death in the United States.

Coronary atherosclerosis may cause the heart to enlarge and weaken the heart muscle until it fails, causing the features of heart failure previously mentioned. It may affect electrical activity and rhythm (discussed in Chapter IV).

Complete, thorough medical examinations by the most competent heart specialists may yield normal findings only a matter of hours or days before the fateful heart attack occurs, because the doctor does not have adequate tools to provide sufficient information about the state of the coronary arteries. With advanced X-ray procedures, it is possible to inject dye into the large coronary arteries and note the presence or absence of obstructions. Evidence of atherosclerosis, however, doesn't tell you when a plaque is going to rupture into the lumen of the artery. The self-assurance that one often feels after having a complete medical examination isn't always warranted. Most medical examinations are effective in a negative way, that is by detecting the presence of disease rather than excluding it. We do know, however, the general factors associated with an increased risk for heart attacks. The great killer's battle plan is known.

The immediate cause of a heart attack is an inadequate blood supply to an area of the ventricle causing damage and destruction of muscle fibers. The blood supply to an area of the heart muscle may be suddenly obstructed by a clot or thrombus in one of the coronary arteries. Despite the coronary occlusion caused by the clot, if there is sufficient blood supply through other arteries, muscle damage may not occur. Preceding the formation of the thrombus in the coronary artery, atherosclerosis develops in the arterial wall and damages the intima, or inner lining. It is this damaged arterial wall that incites nature's normal repair mechanism in the bloodstream to begin clot formation.

There are three factors that are primarily responsible for the atherosclerosis in the artery wall. One of these is the abnormal fat content in the bloodstream—specifically high levels of blood cholesterol and beta-lipoproteins with abnormal cholesterol-phospholipid ratios. The more fat particles that migrate through the arterial wall, the greater likelihood that some will precipitate out in the vessel wall, starting the formation of the atheromatous plaque. The fat deposits in the vessel wall have essentially the same composition as the beta-lipoproteins. There are many factors which may influence the level of blood fats. Regardless of which one or ones are at fault, the blood fat abnormality is a major factor in increasing coronary atherosclerosis.

A second factor is the level of blood pressure. The migration of fat particles from the bloodstream outward through the arterial wall is markedly influenced by the pressure inside the vessel. The higher the pressure the more fat particles will be pushed outward. In this way, a relatively average blood-cholesterol value may still be associated with atherosclerosis if the blood pressure is very high. On the other hand, if the blood pressure is very low increased levels of blood cholesterol are less apt to cause atherosclerosis.

A third factor is the character of the vessel wall—in other words, whether it is fertile soil for planting or retaining the fat particles. A damaged vessel wall, whether it is from inflammation, mechanical or nutritional factors, appears to be more receptive to the deposition of fatty particles. This helps to explain the presence of localized disease in certain arteries in the body. It is possible that the characteristics of the arterial walls in some individuals are less receptive to deposition of fat particles and in some way offer a degree of protection against atherosclerosis. Clearly, all three of these factors are important in the formation of coronary atherosclerosis. Abnormalities of all three factors multiply the probability of having a heart attack.

Behind the three major mechanisms in producing atherosclerosis there is a host of other factors which may influence them. Heredity is a factor, but one can't do much about choosing his parents. It is true that sex is a factor. The male of the species is far more susceptible to the development of atherosclerosis. There is some evidence that different body types—whether one is a long, skinny runner type or the weight-lifter type—may have some association with atherosclerosis. There is always the question of variations in the anatomy of the coronary arteries as an accident of birth. None of these secondary factors is likely to be controlled.

Most of the factors which relate to the role of blood pressure, blood cholesterol, and arterial wall are within the range of control. It is appreciated that inadequate levels of exercise are associated with an increased incidence of atherosclerosis and heart attacks. This effect may be mediated through the influence of exercise on blood fat particles or through its influence in augmenting the number and size of arterial connections to provide blood flow to the heart muscle, by influencing the character and strength of the heart muscle itself, and, finally, by helping to control body weight. Clearly, the level of exercise is something which can be controlled.

As noted in the chapter on Food, Fat, and Fate, dietary factors are exceptionally important. The dietary changes which might be necessary to affect favorably the blood-cholesterol level may differ between individuals, but one can control calorie intake, avoid saturated fats and concentrated carbohydrates, while maintaining an appropriate intake of vitamins (specifically including vitamin C), essential nutrients, and poly-unsaturated fats.

Body weight is clearly a factor which influences the likelihood of a heart attack. Increased body weight is often associated with increased blood pressure. It is also a common factor in the abnormal elevation of blood cholesterol. In a significant number of moderately overweight, middle-aged American males, elevated blood pressure, elevated blood cholesterol, and abnormal blood sugar studies similar to that in diabetes are all reversible with significant reduction of dangerous fat deposits. Excess body fat increases the work of the heart. The heart muscle of a fat man must receive more blood through the coronary arteries to accomplish many of the same physical tasks that can be done with a lesser amount of blood flow to the heart muscle in trim individuals. The fat is merely a weight pack.

The man who is a heavy cigarette smoker may increase the likelihood of a heart attack threefold. Clearly, cigarette smoking is something that is within our control. Certain endocrine and metabolic disorders, such as diabetes, diseases of the adrenal gland, and abnormally low function of the thyroid all contribute to atherosclerosis. Some of these abnormalities of metabolism significantly increase the levels of blood fat and certain of them, such as diabetes, may have an influence on the arterial wall. Their influence in producing atherosclerosis can be significantly affected by proper medical management.

Finally, there is the question of stress. Certainly in susceptible individuals, stress can increase the level of blood cholesterol, at least on a transitory basis. By permitting the accumulation in the heart muscle of products secreted by the adrenal gland, the heart's efficient use of oxygen may be impaired. As a result, even the heart muscle, while the person is at rest, needs more oxygen and more coronary blood flow. Stress may be an important factor, but its effects on the heart in the development of atherosclerosis may be severely blunted by an appropriate exercise program, proper diet, prevention of excess body fat, and the development of an appropriate habit mechanism to eliminate cigarettes or excessive use of stimulants and alcohol.

Who then has coronary atherosclerosis? The battle plan of the great killer gives him many opportunities to strike, but the vast majority of his victims in the American population are the overfed, underfit smokers. Any one of these factors discussed can be associated with an increased risk of heart disease; but if you combine several of them, the likelihood of having a heart attack is increased manifold. In some, the heart attack will appear as a silent episode; in others, the first evidence of the great killer's presence will be sudden death. The lucky ones will make it to the hospital, and of these twenty to forty per cent will not survive.

The Silent Heart Attack

You can have a heart attack and never know it. Estimates differ but studies directed toward determining how often silent heart attacks occur suggest that at least one-third of all heart attacks occur without significant indication. A person may feel nothing at all, or he may have a few days of fatigue or very mild nausea—symtoms mild enough not to stimulate a visit to the doctor. Periodic examinations of young flying crews in the United States Air Force proved that on one examination the electrocardiogram and other elements of the examination might be entirely normal, while on a subsequent examination the electrocardiographic changes associated with a heart attack were unmistakably present. Often these individuals had not had any illness whatsoever.

Autopsy studies frequently demonstrate evidence of old heart attacks in patients without a record of heart disease. Most silent heart attacks are identified on the basis of electrocardiographic changes or by autopsy examinations. Apparently silent infarcts fail to damage a sufficient quantity of muscle to impair seriously the heart's normal pumping action. Most of these individuals probably did not engage in any unusual physical activity that required a major work effort by their heart at the time the infarction occurred. Some cases identified in the Air Force study by electrocardiograms had been recent attacks. The electrocardiogram was still showing progressive changes from a heart attack, unknown to the patients.

The true silent heart attack does not precipitate any adverse reflex behavior which would cause an abnormality in the beating of the heart, fainting, or shocklike episodes that sometimes accompany heart attacks.

There are some individuals who have occlusion of a coronary artery but no apparent muscle damage. Presumably, these individuals have enough blood supply through other blood vessels to the heart muscle to prevent muscle damage. The frequent occurrence of silent infarctions is one of the reasons for regular periodic medical examinations, which should include an electrocardiogram.

Because electrocardiograms have their own individual variations, somewhat like fingerprints, every individual should have an electrocardiogram in early adult life. Such records form useful baselines for detecting significant changes that help to identify the problem of coronary atherosclerosis. Early identification of individual variations, which mimic changes caused by heart disease, may prevent an erroneous diagnosis from causing needless worries, difficulties in obtaining life insurance, and many other complications to the normal course of life.

Sudden Death

Once again the base was on alert. The Strategic Air Command crews were standing by in the ready room, awaiting the signal to prepare for an enemy attack. Some of the men were playing cards, others played pool, most drank Cokes and smoked cigarettes. It would have felt good to take a long walk, play a game of golf, or do anything a little more active, but they had gotten used to waiting —waiting for the signal. Suddenly the signal came; cards were thrown down, Coke bottles dropped, and cue sticks left on the table. The men scrambled for the aircraft. A young pilot clambered aboard his jet aircraft and taxied down the runway. Suddenly his aircraft began to slow down, gradually coasted off its course, and careened into another parked aircraft. Men rushed to the side of the jet to see what had happened. Inside, the young man sat slumped over his controls—he was dead. The enemy had claimed the young Air Force pilot, but the enemy was not a plane from a hostile nation—it was coronary atherosclerosis.

The most common cause of death in young men is coronary artery disease. A large portion of the half-million people a year who die from heart attacks never make it to the hospital. When they get to the hospital they are dead on arrival—D.O.A. Coronary care units, artificial hearts, transplanted hearts, and medical miracles are of no help to these people. By the time they get to the hospital, it is already too late. An appreciable number of these individuals could be salvaged if more people from the general population were trained in providing artificial support for the heart and circulation. Immediate efforts to support the circulation might well have saved this young pilot's life—cheating atherosclerosis of its easy victory. Of course, the American diet, the restricted activity of the ready room, the cokes, the cigarettes, the peak physical exertion associated with the sudden dash to the airplane, all have the familiar ring of the pathway to atherosclerosis.

The Fleeting Heart Pain

Since heart attacks can be either silent or cause severe incapacitating pain, it should be obvious that a wide spectrum of different pains of varying duration, character, and location can be caused by coronary atherosclerosis. While some chest pain is rather typical and easily diagnosed, many other episodes require the skill of a physician to accurately identify their cause. Anyone having chest pain should seek medical advice. It is important to realize, however, that *not all heart pain is in the chest and not all chest pain is caused by the heart.* Chest pain can be caused from a variety of disorders—from indigestion to sore chest muscles. Some forms of chest discomfort are related to apprehension. Sorting out these complexities is what the doctor is for.

The typical fleeting chest pain of coronary atherosclerosis is called angina pectoris, meaning "strangulation of the breastbone." An episode might more appropriately be described as a sensation rather than a pain. Some individuals feel as if a vise is tightening around their chest or a tight band is constricting the thorax. Others describe the sensation as one of a fist knotted up underneath the breastbone (sternum). It may be described as a pressure sensation. The episode is often accompanied with a sensation of impending death.

The location of the discomfort is usually in the center of the chest. It may radiate to the pit of the stomach, upward into the throat, or to the left of the mid-breast directly over the heart.

The discomfort may radiate into the jaw, or sometimes into the left shoulder, and down the left arm. Less often, the discomfort may extend into the right shoulder and right arm. Variations of this discomfort may be noted in different people. In one person most of it may appear to be in the pit of the stomach; in others the discomfort may be localized in the jaw; some may note the discomfort only in the arm and shoulder. It is almost never exclusively located below and to the left of the left nipple, or radiated to the back. The pressure and aching sensation differs in severity. In some individuals it is a fleeting momentary disturbance, in others it is a violent sense of pain. The person may become pale with an almost shocklike appearance.

A constant feature of fleeting heart pain is its short duration. To be properly classified as angina pectoris, the pain should last "less than a quarter of an hour." Most episodes are of much shorter duration. Within moments after the episode has begun, it ceases. Typical pain of longer duration is more often associated with damage to the heart muscle.

Individuals who have recurrent episodes of fleeting heart pain soon learn the factors that cause them. Some attacks are precipitated by anger or severe emotion. One early medical writer, who experienced recurrent episodes, noted its relationship to anger. He wrote that whoever could anger him held his life in his hand, and indeed he died during a fit of anger. Fleeting heart pain may be caused by physical exertion. A hill which an individual may have climbed all his life may become associated with episodes of heart pain. The individual learns how much work he can do without developing chest discomfort. Exposure to cold may precipitate transitory heart pain—particularly while walking into a cold wind. Heavy meals may be a precipitating factor. The combination of a recent meal with physical exertion may be the necessary triggering mechanism. Occasionally individuals are sensitive to tobacco. They learn that continuing the smoking habit is to invite continual recurrence of chest discomfort.

The pattern of angina pectoris changes with the course of time. In some individuals attacks begin to occur spontaneously; in others, smaller and smaller amounts of physical activity will precipitate the episodes. In its most severe form, recurrent episodes occur during bed rest or one may be awakened from sleep with pain. Body weight, blood pressure, associated damage to the valves of the heart, and the extent of coronary atherosclerosis all combine to affect the course and pattern of fleeting heart pain called angina pectoris.

Between attacks of fleeting heart pain, an individual may be entirely normal. A complete thorough physical examination may not reveal a single abnormality. Some of these individuals appear to be in robust health. Extensive laboratory studies are all normal and even the electrocardiographic tracing is often normal. The physician must rely heavily upon the story of the disorder presented by the patient. If the opportunity exists to obtain an electrocardiogram during an attack, characteristic changes may be seen. These subside soon after the discomfort has passed. The fact that a person can have a completely normal medical examination and still have enough undetectable heart disease to cause recurrent pain is sufficient testimony concerning the inadequacy of present-day medical examinations in defining the presence or absence of disease inside the body. While medical examinations have shown marked improvement through the years, in the case of heart disease it still requires a medical Sherlock Holmes to make a correct diagnosis.

Women are more apt to have angina pectoris than men. In either sex, the onset of fleeting heart pains in a person without damaged heart valves or heart defects caused by birth, usually means that occlusion of a coronary artery has occurred. The relatively short duration and nature of the pain suggests that the heart muscle has not been significantly damaged. Nevertheless, nature's redundant system in supplying blood to the heart muscle is severely compromised. The amount of blood available to the heart muscle is limited to the extent that any increased requirements of the heart can cause transitory heart pain.

A Painful Heart Attack

It is the individual with a painful heart attack who is admitted to the hospital—if he lives long enough. Within the hospital, the victim often hovers between life and death for two or three weeks, while loved ones wait to see if he will be one of the lucky ones who survive. The painful heart attack is associated with damage to the large left ventricle muscle responsible for pumping blood to all of the body except the lungs. Unfortunately, in any one person it is not possible to predict when, if ever, he will have a heart attack.

The painful heart attack may strike without warning at any time. At the end of a scrumptious dinner, a gradual fullness may increase in the pit of the stomach until it is a pressure sensation in the lower central chest, or actual nausea and vomiting may ensue. The dull, constricting pain similar to that noted in fleeting heart pain may make itself known during any activity or during any period of rest. Its hallmark is its longer duration. The pain frequently lasts more than fifteen minutes. The discomfort has the same general locations as noted in angina pectoris, often involving the central part of the chest, radiating into the jaw or the arms. The pain may be very severe, causing the individual to feel as if a very heavy weight were resting upon his chest. Often the episode may waken an individual from a deep sleep. The duration and severity of the pain varies markedly, from mild discomfort to a feeling of having been "kicked in the chest by a mule." The more severe discomfort is often associated with anxiety and fear of death. The individual often wants to sit upright, feeling he can get his breath better in the upright position.

Very mild heart pain may produce no significant change in physical appearance. More severe discomfort is often associated with a sudden paleness of the skin. Beads of sweat may pop out upon the forehead and eventually the whole body may be drenched with light perspiration. The pale, anxious individual with a sweaty face and his hand resting over the front of his chest, is typical of the individual having an acute heart attack.

The blood pressure may either rise or fall. Acute injury of the heart may cause severe constriction of the small arteries with a marked rise in blood pressure. This increases the work of the heart even more, although the heart muscle is already having difficulty. Sometimes the distal arteries dilate excessively through a reflex mechanism. This can cause profound weakness or even loss of consciousness. In its severe form it is the "shock" of a heart attack. The shock itself requires treatment and is an indication that the road to recovery will be a rocky one.

The shock reaction accompanying an acute painful heart attack may be completely out of proportion to the amount of damage to the heart muscle. Small amounts of damage or threats to the body can change the heart and circulation mechanism in a way to produce shock. A good example of this is a case in which simple needle puncture to draw a small blood sample may set off a reflex reaction in a sensitive individual that causes a severe faint, or a form of shock. The amount of tissue damage or injury to the individual is almost nonexistent. So it is with an acute heart attack, even the smallest amount of muscle damage can set off powerful reflexes that tend to slow or nearly stop the heart or cause the terminal arteries to dilate excessively. Either one or the combination of these effects causes a precipitous fall in blood pressure. The skin often becomes a pale chalky color. If the shocklike reaction of a heart attack is not associated with severe heart muscle damage, an individual can recover from shock and still have a good strong heart with little or no residual evidence of muscle damage.

The acute, painful heart attack can cause heart failure by damaging the heart muscle. The physician often hears changes in breath sounds, caused by an accumulation of small amounts of fluid in the lungs. Minimal damage to the heart muscle may not affect its pumping ability and not cause heart failure. The more extensive the damage to the heart muscle, the more likely severe heart failure will develop. When this occurs, the entire gamut of events associated with heart failure can occur.

Damaged heart muscle may cause irregularities of the heartbeat. Some of these are of minor consequence while others are of great importance. The development of sporadic extra beats from the ventricle suggests that the damaged heart muscle is electrically unstable. Early detection of this tendency and the administration of the appropriate medicines can prevent the development of more serious irregularities of the heart. All too often the irregularity of the heart is the sudden occurrence of the rhythm of death. The immediate recognition of such an irregularity, followed by prompt treatment, is one purpose for the "coronary care units" that have sprung up over the nation.

Coronary care units provide constant observation twenty-four hours a day, for a variable period of time, to detect any evidence of electrical instability of the heart that requires immediate attention. Small units to provide acute intensive care for individuals admitted to the hospital with new heart attacks have significantly improved the chances of survival for the hospitalized individual. The major accomplishment of these units has been to provide around-the-clock observation of the characteristics of the heartbeat. Trained nursing personnel and available physicians institute immediate action when electrical instability of the heart is noted. If the rhythm of death (ventricular fibrillation) occurs, these individuals are trained to provide immediate support to the heart in maintaining its pumping action and correcting the beating of the heart immediately. These procedures must be initiated within a matter of minutes. When the heart stops pumping effectively, brain damage or death is usually less than four minutes away. The sooner adequate circulation can be restored, the less likely it is that there will be significant damage to the brain or other vital organs.

Coronary care units have been established at Cornell's New York Hospital, Massachusetts General Hospital, Boston's Peter Bent Brigham Hospital, and other major hospitals throughout the country with varied degrees of success. In almost every instance, the number of deaths from acute heart attacks in patients admitted to the unit has been decreased by at least half. In some of the more experienced units, death from irregularities of the heart has become almost nonexistent. Many individuals who have had the rhythm of death have lived to tell about it and returned to useful, productive lives with little or no limitation on their activities.

Not all hospital facilities have coronary care units. As an interested citizen, you should find out if your available hospital facility does or does not have one. If not, your chances of surviving an acute heart attack, should you live long enough to be admitted to the hospital, are decreased by at least fifty per cent. Around-the-clock special nurses, constantly at the bedside of the patient with modern instruments available to register continuously the characteristics of the heartbeat, can go a long way toward providing the same support as a coronary care unit. In essence, such a situation is a small coronary care unit for one patient. The absence of equipment to observe continually the characteristics of the heartbeat or the absence of trained personnel, or the absence of suitable emergency equipment immediately at the bedside, provides an opportunity for the rhythm of death to occur suddenly without previous warning, with no one present with the appropriate medicines or equipment to restore the heartbeat to normal. The absence of good coronary care units in many hospitals throughout the United States is a direct result of inadequate funds available for the relatively expensive specialized equipment and the lack of available trained personnel.

Some information concerning the amount of damaged heart muscle can be obtained by blood analysis. Certain enzymes released from the damaged heart muscle fibers are an indicator of the infarcted muscle. These and other changes in the blood are confirmatory evidence of heart muscle damage. During healing many of the values return to previous levels.

Another aid in identifying an acute heart attack and following its progress, is the electrocardiogram. Not all individuals will show typical electrical changes on the heart tracing, but usually the changes will be very helpful in identifying the heart attack and its effect upon the heart muscle. Certain characteristics of the heart tracing return toward normal during recovery. Residual changes in the heart tracing may persist for years after a heart attack.

Since infarction of the heart muscle is caused by an inadequate blood supply to part of it, everything possible should be done during this critical phase to eliminate any increased demand for blood flow to the heart muscle. In short, the heart needs a rest. The work of the heart should be limited as much as possible to minimize its oxygen requirements and the need for blood flow. This, of course, is the reason for strict rest during a new heart attack.

Most heart specialists agree concerning the need for rest for the heart during this critical phase. There are differences of opinion concerning how best to provide rest for the heart. Not too many years ago, when a person was admitted to the hospital with a new heart attack, he stayed in bed a minimum of six weeks. Bed rest in those days really meant bed rest. Usually the bed was kept absolutely level. The individual was not allowed to sit up or prop himself up on the pillow. For weeks the sheets on his bed were changed by rolling the patient from side to side. Often the patient was not allowed to brush his teeth or even feed himself. Eventually, if he was allowed to read, a bed stand was rolled up to the proper distance and someone else turned the pages of the magazine or book for him. More often than not, someone else read to him. After the period of hospitalization from a new heart attack, these individuals were often doomed to a life of invalidism.

In more recent years, this concept has been challenged and it is a rare occasion to see an individual with a new heart attack treated in such a severe manner. Unless the individual is in shock or has other problems with his circulation that would make it inadvisable, many heart specialists now have their patients sit up in bed and others may even have them sit in a chair beside the bed, soon after the initial pain has subsided. There does not appear to be any significant increased work effort on the heart when one is seated upright as opposed to lying in bed. The column of blood in the aorta above the heart, in the upright position, provides an increased pressure head for filling of the coronary arteries when the heart muscle is relaxed during diastole. In this sense, the seated position may offer some advantages in providing adequate blood flow to the damaged heart muscle.

Some heart specialists feel that the ability to sit up in bed or a chair, and less severe restrictions on activity, provide such an additional bonus in relieving anxiety, that the net result provides better rest for the heart and circulation. Since excitement and emotion do increase the work of the heart, immediately after a recent heart attack the number of visitors or other possible emotional stimuli is usually limited.

Many common aspects of everyday living must be evaluated in terms of decreasing the load on the heart. These efforts include special diets when food is allowed in the course of the illness and attention to whether certain stimulating drinks such as coffee should be permitted. The care of the bowels becomes increasingly important. A previously active individual who is suddenly hospitalized can easily become constipated. This situation is aggravated in the presence of a heart attack because certain commonly used medicines have a constipating effect. Unless attention is given to this matter, three to four days after the attack, an accumulated hard bowel movement has to be passed. This is at the exact critical time when the newly damaged heart muscle is weakest and most apt to rupture. Straining, associated with a difficult bowel movement, is an all too frequent cause for a "blowing out" of the heart muscle, leading to instantaneous death. These problems are usually prevented by proper bowel management.

Passing the hurdle of the first bowel movement after a new heart attack is an important signpost. It heralds the beginning of a return to more normal function of the body. To prevent the straining and other problems that can occur with a bowel movement, most heart specialists today prefer to have the patient picked up and set on a commode beside the bed. Shallow bedpans are almost impossible. Expecting an individual to have a bowel movement in such a device, particularly lying down in bed, is to ask a patient to undergo a significant risk. Such an unnatural position for a bowel movement inevitably leads to straining. Heart specialists have long recognized the importance of passing the milestone of the first bowel movement. It was for this reason, and because he knew that all of the individuals in the medical profession would understand its importance, that Dr. Paul Dudley White announced to the world on television when President Eisenhower had his first bowel movement following his heart attack.

A variety of medicines are used by the doctor during the acute heart attack. What medicines are chosen depends upon the nature of the case. If heart failure is present, medicines to help correct this must be used. If there is an irregularity of the heart, other medications can be used for this purpose. If there is a tendency for the heart to beat too slowly or nearly stop, there are medicines for this. If the blood pressure is too low or there is evidence of shock, specific medicines may be used to restore the normal contraction of the terminal arteries. If the blood pressure is too high, other medications may be used to lower it and decrease the work of the heart.

Usually the doctor prescribes medicine to prevent blood clotting. This may prevent the extension and size of the clot in the coronary artery. It is of value in preventing the development of clots in the leg vessels or other veins in the body during periods of inactivity and bed rest. Clots may also form inside the heart, next to the damaged heart muscle, unless such medications are given. Clots in the legs or in the heart may cause sudden death if they are released and escape into the circulation. Clots in the left side of the heart may go to the brain, producing a stroke, or to the kidneys, or to any other artery in the body. Clots in the leg veins can pass through the right heart and directly to the lungs.

Finally, if all has gone well during the critical phase of the heart attack, the time comes when the individual must be prepared to return to more normal living. This is done by gradually increasing the amount of time the individual may sit up, if he has been in bed, then gradually increasing the amount of walking he can do around his hospital room and finally in the hospital corridors. The purpose is to improve gradually the individual's ability to take care of all of his normal functions. Most heart specialists do not make an effort to significantly increase the patient's activity until at least three weeks after the initial heart attack has occurred.

This period of time is needed to form new scar tissue to replace the damaged heart muscle. The healing process in the wall of the ventricle takes time. If too much activity is permitted too soon, a good scar is not formed and poor healing results. Usually a new heart attack closes off a major artery supplying a significant portion of heart muscle. The connections between the terminal branches of this artery and the other major arteries to the heart now become very important. It takes time to develop new blood vessels and increase the capacity of previously existing connections. A period of at least three to five weeks is needed to permit adequate development of new routes to supply blood to the working heart muscle. In most instances, the process will not be complete by then and will continue for several months thereafter. Many factors will influence the adequate development of a new blood supply. These different factors influence whether or not the physical activity of an individual should be increased and how much.

Do You Have High Blood Pressure?

Doctors have long debated what is normal blood pressure. Population surveys have demonstrated a linear relationship between increased blood pressure and increased heart disease—specifically atherosclerosis. Rather than a magic figure, which defines the difference between normal and abnormal blood pressure, the truth is—the higher your blood pressure, the more likely atherosclerosis will develop. One of the features which appears to protect Cleveland's industrialized Navajo Indians from atherosclerosis is a tendency toward low blood pressure. These observations attest to the importance of preventing elevated blood pressure. A wise old physician was once seeing a patient whose blood pressure was relatively low. On previous examinations, the patient had been told that he had "low blood pressure." The old doctor gradually pumped up the blood pressure cuff and recorded his reading. Finally, he turned abruptly to the patient and said, "Do you know what's the first thing you should do when you find out you've got low blood pressure?" The patient replied, "Why, no, Doctor." Whereupon the wise old physician said, "Go home, get down on your knees and thank God you've got it!"

What is labile blood pressure? There are a number of individuals who intermittently exhibit high blood pressure values. These elevations in blood pressure are usually transitory. They can occur with stress or even the apprehension of a medical examination. Persistence in examining these people usually demonstrates that the blood pressure fluctuates wildly but during periods of rest with adequate reassurance, it may return to much lower levels. Whether or not such marked lability in the blood pressure is dangerous remains a matter of dispute. The real answer probably rests with the degree of elevation and what proportion of the days, weeks, months, or years the blood pressure is significantly elevated. If such elevations are sporadic, occurring for a few minutes two or three times a year, they are not likely to have any significant effect on the development of atherosclerosis. The individual chronically exposed to stress, with persistent marked elevations of blood pressure and only intermittent lower values throughout his working day, has ample opportunity to develop atherosclerosis.

What Causes Elevated Blood Pressure?

Control of the blood pressure is a very complex matter. The blood pressure depends upon the resistance offered by the arteries to the blood pumped by the heart. If the cardiac output falls, the blood pressure falls. When the resistance in the arteries is diminished for example by dilating the terminal arteries, the blood pressure falls, even though the cardiac output is unchanged. If the cardiac output stays the same and the terminal arteries are constricted, the blood pressure rises. These fundamental relationships are not in dispute and are well understood. The influence of excitement or exercise in augmenting cardiac output is a good example of how blood pressure may be elevated. The less well understood aspects of blood pressure are the factors which increase the cardiac output or cause constriction. If the blood volume is increased, this can raise the blood pressure. More recently, some investigators have identified small tumors in the adrenal gland that secrete hormones, which influence the constriction of the arteries and cardiac output to cause increased blood pressure. These small tumors are spotted throughout the external part of the adrenal gland and may play a significant role in elevated blood pressure in many individuals in whom no cause could previously be demonstrated. The methods of identifying this abnormality in the adrenal gland as a cause for elevated blood pressure are somewhat complex, but they are being simplified, and the time is not too far off when individuals with this problem can be readily identified and treated. A very uncommon type of tumor in the center of the adrenal gland has long been recognized as a cause for increased blood pressure.

For years the kidney has been implicated as a cause for elevated blood pressure. In some instances, by releasing certain hormones into the bloodstream, the kidney can act like an endocrine gland and cause constriction of the arteries. The kidney usually does this when its own blood supply is limited. Atherosclerosis in the arteries to the kidneys can and does cause elevated blood pressure. If the disease is localized outside the kidney, the obstruction can sometimes be removed. If only one kidney is involved while the other one is perfectly normal, in some cases removal of the abnormal kidney causes blood pressure to return to normal.

Many people have elevated blood pressure with no apparent cause. Unless a correctable problem of the adrenal gland or in the kidneys is identified, the physician usually is left with the alternative of symptomatic treatment. He uses medications directed toward lowering the blood pressure to a more acceptable level or preventing the complications that may result from persistently ele vated blood pressure.

When constriction of the terminal arteries causes increased blood pressure, the work of the heart is increased. Each time the heart pumps blood into the aorta, it must do it with greater force. The increased contraction of the heart muscle increases its demands and needs for oxygen. In the course of time this leads to increased strength and size of the heart muscle, or cardiac enlargement. Initially, the size of the ventricular cavity may not be increased. The wall of the left ventricle gradually increases in thickness and strength, much like a weight lifter's muscle. Essentially, high blood pressure causes the left ventricle to be a weight-lifting muscle. The X-ray shadow of the heart may not show any significant increase in size at this stage. Later on, as a mechanism to increase its efficiency, if the left ventricle dilates, evidence of this can be seen in the X-ray. Long-standing high blood pressure also produces changes in the electrocardiogram. The voltage generated by the enlarged heart muscle is increased. Other changes in the wave form may develop in the course of time.

Why Is High Blood Pressure Dangerous?

Until the relationship of increased blood pressure to athero-sclerosis was more clearly understood, a prevailing opinion among heart specialists was that you didn't treat blood pressure—you treated the complications when they occurred. The simple truth is that the major complications of high blood pressure are almost without exception caused by atherosclerosis. The elevated blood pressure can cause atherosclerosis in the arteries to the brain. These damaged arteries, under increased pressure, may be occluded by a clot or they may rupture. Either event will produce a stroke. The stroke is a complication of the atherosclerotic process which can be accelerated by elevated blood pressure. In a similar manner, many individuals with high blood pressure have heart attacks. This is directly related to the increase in atherosclerosis in the coronary arteries. The increased work imposed upon the left ventricular muscle and the problems associated with atherosclerotic coronary arteries may lead to left heart failure. Progressive atherosclerosis in the arteries to the kidneys eventually leads to failure of these organs.

The lesson to be learned is, high blood pressure, regardless of its cause, creates its damaging effect by accelerating atherosclerosis. For this reason, not only is it important to utilize available measures to control the blood pressure, but it is equally important to eliminate those factors which also contribute to atherosclerosis. In short, the individual with high blood pressure has an added incentive to control his body weight to prevent the accumulation of dangerous fat deposits, use a non-atherosclerotic diet, and avoid cigarette smoking. If atherosclerosis could be prevented in the presence of high blood pressure, most individuals could live with the increased pressure without significant difficulty. In fact, many women forty years of age or less, who have relatively severe elevated blood pressure, may live reasonably normal life-spans because of their protection against atherosclerosis until later in life than men. It should be noted, however, that women with high blood pressure develop atherosclerotic changes much earlier than women with lower blood pressure. One of the causes for heart attacks in young women is persistently elevated blood pressure.

Stenosis of the Mitral Valve

In order for the four-chambered heart to be an effective pump all of its valves must be normal. Abnormalities in the mitral valve can limit the effectiveness of the heart pump. With the decrease in rheumatic fever, mitral valve disease is now less common in the United States. When the mitral valve, resting between the great left atrial reservoir and the inlet into the left ventricular cavity, becomes narrowed and obstructed (stenosed) it is called *mitral stenosis*. This is usually caused by inflammation of the two valve cusps. Gradually scar tissue forms across the leaflets, sealing their edges together, causing the valve opening to become smaller and smaller. Normally, in the adult, the valve opening will admit two or three fingers, but with mitral stenosis the opening may be as small as the diameter of a cigarette.

Occasionally, individuals who have been living active lives, such as are required with regular military duty, are found with severe obstruction to the mitral valve, obviously present for many years without being recognized. With severe obstruction, changes occur in the heart and eventually cause difficulties.

The obstruction between the left aterial and left ventricular cavity literally dams up blood in the left atrium. The pressure inside the left atrium increases and causes it to enlarge. The elevated pressure is transmitted backward into the lungs, just as occurs in left heart failure. The lungs become engorged with blood, which may be demonstrated by X-ray studies. Finally, these large dilated vessels in the lungs may erode into the windpipe or its branches, causing such individuals to cough up blood—sometimes as the first indication of underlying disease. Many individuals notice a gradual onset of shortness of breath, caused by excessive accumulation of blood in the lungs.

Engorgement of the lungs tends to impede the flow of blood from the right ventricle to the lungs; consequently the pressure in the right ventricle gradually increases, causing the right heart to enlarge. Enlargement of the left atrium and the right heart is often detected by electrocardiographic and X-ray studies. A cardiac catheterization may be performed, which consists of slipping a small hollow tube through a vein in the arm or leg and gradually advancing it into the right atrium. The tube is then passed on through the right ventricle and out through the pulmonary artery into the lung field following the course of circulation. It may be wedged out into the smallest branch of the pulmonary artery. Here, the increased pressure backed up from the left atrium may be measured. Increased pressure in the pulmonary artery and right ventricle may be noted as the hollow catheter is withdrawn. These and other complex studies enable the doctor to assess the amount of obstruction being caused by the diseased mitral valve.

While the left atrium and the right heart are working to overcome the obstruction at the mitral valve area, the left ventricle is spared. It is more difficult for the left atrium to load the left ventricle with blood, since it must squeeze the blood past the narrow orifice opening into the left ventricle. As a result, the left ventricle may be smaller than seen in normal individuals. Occasionally, calcification and disease of the mitral valve extends into part of the heart muscle and acts as a splint against the movement of the muscle itself. This further diminishes the ability of the left ventricular muscle to act as an efficient pump. Mitral stenosis may limit the amount of blood that can be pumped by the left ventricle to the body. Relieving the obstruction caused by the scarring which joined the two valve leaflets together, either by tearing them or cutting them, was one of the earliest successful heart operations. The procedure has been perfected in the last twenty years. Release of the obstruction was usually associated with a marked improvement in the function of the heart. Since open heart surgery became possible, badly diseased valves are now cut out and replaced by mechanical valves.

Mitral Valve Leak

Occasionally the two leaflets of the mitral valve do not meet properly, providing incomplete closure of the opening between the left atrium and the left ventricle. Small openings do not have any major effect on the pumping action of the heart. With large defects a great deal of blood may be squirted backward into the left atrial cavity rather than out into the aorta when the left ventricular muscle contracts. This condition is called *mitral insufficiency*. A common cause for this defect is rheumatic fever. Inflammation of the valve results in scarring and retraction of its edges until they do not close properly. In this instance, the left ventricle is not spared. The left ventricular cavity must fill with extra blood during diastole. In addition to the normal stroke volume ejected into the aorta, extra blood regurgitates back into the left atrial cavity. In severe mitral insufficiency, constant, massive regurgitation into the left atrium leads to its progressive enlargement and dilatation. The atrium may stretch and distend until it occupies almost the entire width of the chest. In such conditions the large left atrial reservoir looks like a huge washtub.

Unless there is an associated obstruction of the mitral valve, the pulmonary engorgement seen with mitral stenosis does not occur with leakage of the valve. Eventually the overworked left ventricle fails. The increasing pressure in the left atrium causes respiratory symptoms, including accumulation of fluid in the lungs. Many individuals live with a moderate leakage of the mitral valve throughout a relatively normal life-span without difficulty. As the size of the leak progresses, however, further changes develop, often causing sudden massive left heart failure. In more recent years, as with mitral stenosis, it is possible to replace the damaged valve with an artificial one. Since many individuals live a normal life-span with a minimal leak, major surgery of this type is not indicated unless the defect is severe and the evidence is convincing that the subsequent course will be rapidly downhill. Artificial valves cause problems. Medicine to prevent blood clots from forming is usually needed and some valves cause continual destruction of red blood cells, resulting in anemia. There is much room for improvement in mechanical heart valves.

Stenosis of the Aortic Valve

Occasionally the three-cusp aortic valve at the outlet of the heart becomes scarred and stuck together. The condition, *aortic stenosis,* progresses slowly until severe obstruction to the ejection of blood from the left heart into the aorta occurs. The obstruction obviously increases the work of the left ventricular muscle. The overworked muscle enlarges in size and increases its strength. Interestingly enough, individuals with obstruction to the outflow of the left ventricle frequently develop very large coronary arteries, with extensive connections between the terminal arterial branches. Enlargement of the left ventricle can be seen by chest X-ray. Increased voltage and other changes occur in the electrocardiogram. Eventually the left heart fails, followed by a rapidly downhill course. Individuals with aortic stenosis may have sudden unexpected irregularities of the heart, causing immediate death.

In aortic stenosis, the blood pressure in the arm is usually low because the obstruction is between the left ventricle and the arterial tree. The pressure measured by a catheter inside the left ventricular cavity is markedly elevated compared to the pressure in the aorta.

When atherosclerosis of the coronary arteries complicates aortic stenosis, or when the heart muscle becomes too large for its blood supply, myocardial infarction can occur.

A very mild obstruction of the aortic valve may not cause any significant difficulties. Some individuals with mild defects have been able to do strenuous exercise.

In the presence of severe aortic stenosis, the valve today may be replaced surgically. Like all current mechanical valves, however, there are certain disadvantages. The surgery alone is not without considerable risk to life.

Aortic Valve Leak

Inflammation and infection may partially destroy the leaflets of the aortic valve (*aortic insufficiency*), permitting regurgitation of blood into the left ventricular cavity during diastole. The leaky aortic valve decreases the efficiency of the left ventricular muscle in pumping blood forward into the aorta. The more blood that leaks backward into the left ventricle, the greater will be the decrease in efficiency. To illustrate the problem, if the heart must provide 75 ml of blood with each beat for circulation to the body, and if the valve leaks 75 ml back into the left ventricle, the heart must eject 150 ml of blood into the aorta—75 ml for the body and 75 ml for the leak. The leaky aortic valve causes a marked increase in the volume of blood in the left ventricular cavity, and early enlargement of the left ventricle.

The large volume of blood which must be ejected into the aorta causes a sharp rise in systolic blood pressure. In place of a normal value of approximately 125 mmHg, the systolic pressure may be 170 or 200 mmHg (comparable to that observed in normal people during vigorous exercise). With a big leak, blood flows rapidly back into the left ventricle, allowing the diastolic pressure to fall below usual normal values. Instead of a usual value of approximately 70 mmHg, the pressure may drop to 30 mmHg or even 0 mmHg.

The principal effect of an aortic valve leak is to increase the work of the left ventricular muscle. If the leak is small, the increased work requirements may be minimal. I have seen individuals with this defect who were able to exercise to the same levels achieved by pentathletes in training for the Olympic games. The significance of aortic insufficiency literally depends upon the size of the leak. A large leak eventually causes left heart failure. If heart failure cannot be adequately controlled by medicine, eventually consideration must be given to replacing the leaky valve. Many individuals can live to a ripe old age with aortic insufficiency. One out of five having surgery for valve replacement may not survive the operation. The ratio varies with the skill of the surgeon and his honesty in reporting success or failure.

Defects of the Tricuspid Valve

The tricuspid valve between the right atrial reservoir and the right ventricular cavity is less often damaged than the valves in the left heart. The tricuspid valve cusps do not close properly when the right ventricle dilates from heart failure. This, in turn, will cause regurgitation of blood into the right atrium and abnormalities in venous pulsations in the neck and liver. Rarely, the valve may be damaged from rheumatic fever or it may be obstructed as a birth defect.

Pulmonary Valve Defects

Almost all defects of the pulmonary valve are birth defects. If the valve or outlet from the right heart is obstructed it increases the work of the right ventricular muscle. The X-ray and electrocardiogram provide evidence of right heart enlargement. If the obstruction is severe, eventually right heart failure with the usual findings develops. Obstruction to the pulmonary valve or outlet of the right ventricle can usually be corrected by surgical procedures.

Rheumatic Fever

In many parts of the world, rheumatic fever and rheumatic heart disease remain a major medical problem. At one time in the

United States, a large number of young children were afflicted with this disease. Large epidemics of the disorder occurred. Although rheumatic fever is still seen in this country, it is now an uncommon disease. Many doctors graduate from medical school and complete specialty training without ever seeing an actual case of rheumatic fever. Only three decades ago, entire small hospitals were devoted to treating young children with rheumatic fever and the heart disease it caused. Large hospital wards of young children with abdomens swollen with fluid, painful joints, and temperature spikes were commonplace. During World War II certain military camps were hit hard with rheumatic fever, prompting wholesale investigations concerning its cause and how it subsequently produced rheumatic heart disease. These extensive studies occurred almost at the same time that antibiotics became available to medicine in significant quantities. The simultaneous occurrence of these two events has nearly wiped out the problem of rheumatic fever. *Theoretically, rheumatic fever and rheumatic heart disease are preventable and could be eradicated entirely.*

Most authorities accept the concept that rheumatic fever is a complication of a *streptococcal* infection. These bacteria are seen in common respiratory infections—usually in the throat and adjacent respiratory passages. The "strep throat" causes enlargement of the glands in the neck and, in severe form, releases toxins that are carried throughout the body. Man's protective mechanisms are designed to develop immunity or resistance to different infections. In the course of developing an immunity to strep infections, the body develops a form of allergy to the toxins and other products created by the infection. This allergic response affects special tissues in the body—those found in the membranes around the joints and the inner surface of the heart, including the heart valves— causing them to become swollen and inflamed.

The usual story of rheumatic fever begins with a sore throat. By studying throat cultures, the strep germ was identified. Shortly after the throat infection has occurred, the allergy-like reaction begins. The child may begin to have recurrent episodes of fever; he may be listless, tired, and lose his appetite. In the colder climates of the world, the reaction is often accompanied by sore and painful joints. The ankles and knees may become swollen, the skin reddened and hot to touch; the child may complain bitterly on movement of the joint. One day the right knee may be involved, and as it subsides the left knee may become involved. In such a way, the different joints are involved at different times, giving rise to the term *migratory polyarthritis*. Various skin rashes and nodules may also be observed in certain patients.

In more temperate climates, the joint findings are not noted as frequently, and the spiking fever and joint pains may never appear. The process may occur silently in the heart while outwardly the child appears perfectly healthy. The joint involvement of children with rheumatic fever in the cold climates as opposed to the warmer climates has given rise to the term *Boston rheumatic fever*. Certainly Boston was one of the major locations in the United States where rheumatic fever with multiple joint involvement reached near epidemic proportions in young children.

Many individuals with no evidence of rheumatic fever are later found to have typical heart murmurs caused by diseased heart valves. Mitral stenosis, mitral insufficiency, aortic stenosis, aortic insufficiency, or any combination of these valvular defects can be caused by rheumatic fever. Despite its subterfuges, the general characteristics of the disease were identified. The strep infection clearly was the culprit. The proper use of penicillin and appropriate antibiotics was the chief method of early eradication of strep infections. This, in turn, prevented the abnormal allergy-like responses and damaged heart valves. Prevention of rheumatic fever eliminates most requirements for heart valve surgery. The simple truth is that the drama of the operating room is often a needless tragic end to inadequate preventive treatment.

Rheumatic heart disease can also cause an allergy-like inflammatory response of the heart muscle. The muscle fibers are weakened, losing their normal contraction ability, and heart failure may occur. This complication of rheumatic fever is usually of limited duration. If the patient survives the critical phase, the heart muscle may recover with no further damage.

In nations where there is adequate control of strep infections, rheumatic fever has practically disappeared. However, there are certain areas of the world in which strep infections are still common and cause a high incidence of rheumatic fever. Anyone with an identified strep throat deserves immediate and proper treatment. The control of strep infections, particularly during the past two decades, is the principle reason for the marked decrease in rheumatic fever in the United States.

Anyone who has experienced one episode of rheumatic fever, particularly if there is indication of heart disease, should be on penicillin therapy, at least until he is twenty-five, and thereafter should receive penicillin therapy for any acute respiratory infection or when surgical or dental procedures of any type are necessary. This can save him from being "the star" in the drama of the operating room.

How Syphilis Affects the Heart

At one time syphilis was a major cause for damage to the aortic valve. The syphilis organisms would evade the wall of the great aorta, just outside the left ventricular chamber, causing an inflammatory reaction that damaged and weakened the aortic wall. The process often caused obstruction to the opening of the coronary arteries extending from the root of the aorta. In this way, syphilis could limit the blood supply to the heart muscle, producing the same problems as coronary atherosclerosis. When the inflammatory reaction was severe, the aorta would dilate into a saclike expansion. The process often extended from the aorta to involve the aortic valve. The valves would become damaged and the aortic ring that seated the valve would dilate. These changes caused marked aortic insufficiency. At one time the major cause of aortic insufficiency was syphilis. Today, the vast majority of cases of aortic insufficiency are complications of rheumatic fever.

Miscellaneously Acquired Heart Diseases

There are a variety of less common forms of heart disease which may be encountered. One of these, called *pericarditis,* which means inflammation of the sac around the heart, may cause chest pain. Usually the pain is sharper than an acute heart attack and is aggravated by breathing or motion. Sometimes pericarditis follows in the wake of a respiratory infection, although it may occur spontaneously with no apparent cause. It may recur after it has apparently been cured. In most instances pericarditis does not leave permanent residual damage, despite the discomfort it causes at the time.

A variety of inflammations and toxins can affect the heart muscle. This includes the toxin liberated from diphtheria. The control of diphtheria in the United States has made diphtheritic inflammation of the heart muscle almost nonexistent. Even acute pneumonia may extend to inflame and irritate the heart muscle. Many diseases known principally to the tropics also cause inflammation of the heart muscle. Whenever an acute inflammatory disease is present, it is well to keep in mind that it may also cause inflammation of the heart. This is true whether the infection is caused by bacteria, viruses, or fungi.

There are a host of other diseases of the body which also affect the circulatory system. An anemia decreases the ability of the bloodstream to carry oxygen and may increase the work of the heart. In very severe anemias this may be sufficiently critical to cause heart failure. In patients with coronary atherosclerosis, the anemia may limit the ability to supply oxygen to the heart muscle, causing angina pectoris or transitory heart pain. Overactivity of the thyroid gland will require increased delivery of oxygen to all of the different tissues. The increased work expected of the heart muscle plus the effect of the increased amounts of thyroid hormone on the heart may significantly increase the work of the heart as well as its electrical irritability. This may cause heart failure or a number of irregularities of the heartbeat. Abnormally low amounts of thyroid hormone decrease the function of most of the cells throughout the body. This may decrease the need of the heart to pump blood to deliver oxygen, but it also accelerates the process of a therosclerosis—speeding up this process in the coronary arteries. Abnormalities of the heart and circulation, secondary to such problems as thyroid disease or anemia, are usually reversible. If the primary medical problem is correctly treated, the heart and circulation will adjust normally.

Pulmonary disease is still a frequent cause for abnormalities in function of the heart and circulation. The high incidence of fibrosis and scarring of the lung tissues often causes increased resistance to pumping blood through the lungs which increases the workload on the right heart. Eventually this may cause right heart failure. Blood clots going from the right heart to the lungs are another common cause for abnormalities in heart function. These may run the gamut from heart failure to irregularities of the heartbeat or actual stopping of the heart.

The Great Imitator

A number of individuals have symptoms which they attribute to their heart and circulation but which are not associated with any identifiable abnormality. Some of these individuals simply have anxiety. There is a great deal of fear of heart disease because it is not properly understood. An imagined heart disease can blight a person's life, producing real discomfort and unhappiness. Some of these individuals experience repeated episodes of faintness or breathlessness. Others may be more aware of extra or skipped beats. A frequent complaint of these people are stabbing pains below the left nipple. Very often these individuals are not capable of significant amounts of physical activity without discomfort. Some of these problems are not too different from those which normal people experience after a severe illness, prolonged bed rest, or other form of inactivity. A marked sudden increase in the level of physical activity far above the level of one's attained capability will sometimes produce this disorder.

Individuals who have these types of complaints should see their physician and accept his advice when he tells them that he cannot find any evidence of significant heart disease. In many instances, correction of living habits, specifically getting rid of the excess use of tobacco and coffee and instituting a proper exercise program, will go a long way toward correcting the problems. Prolonged inactivity and prolonged acute illnesses require a prolonged time to recover. The process may be gradual but if it is steady, most of these problems can be licked.

Palpitation, faintness, and stabbing pains in the chest have been noted frequently in office workers and other white-collar individuals who have been called into the military services during periods of national emergency. Exercise programs given to these young men were frequently far above their normal level of daily activity. When they were pushed too rapidly, they developed problems. Such observations during World War I led the British physician Sir Thomas Lewis to call this problem *soldier's heart disease.*

When one becomes too concerned about a variety of ill-defined pains, it might be well to remember that atherosclerosis often does not make its presence known until a person either has a full-blown heart attack or drops dead. Until that moment, coronary atherosclerosis may cause no obvious limitation of an individual's activities. It is not manifested by a variety of ill-defined stabbing pains, breathlessness, and palpitation.

Birth Defects of the Heart

Even the problem of birth defects of the heart has been significantly reduced with the advances in medicine. The role of diseases of the mother during pregnancy and its effect on the baby are now much better understood. Methods to protect a mother who has been exposed to German measles are now available, and new vaccines have been developed to insure that the mother will not have other infectious illnesses during pregnancy that could influence the health of her baby. Even new methods have been developed to diagnose and treat the baby in the uterus. These advances in knowledge have tended to decrease the frequency of birth defects of the heart.

In addition to developing methods to decrease the frequency of birth defects of the heart, the ability to operate inside the heart has made it possible in many instances for the surgeon to correct the structural abnormalities caused by birth defects. Not all defects can be corrected, but most of the common ones can be.

A frequent birth defect is the persistence of an arterial shunt between the pulmonary artery and the great aorta (*patent ductus arteriosus*). This arterial shunt is normally present in the fetus during its developmental stage. It enables the heart to shunt the blood through the heart without sending it to the collapsed lungs. Normally, this communication closes at birth, separating the right and left circulation and forcing all of the blood leaving the right heart to go to the lungs for oxygenation. After birth, the pressure in the great aortic artery is much greater than the pressure in the pulmonary artery. If the fetal shunt does not close off when the baby is born, soon thereafter some blood is shunted from the aorta into the pulmonary artery. The shunted blood makes another trip to the lungs, then returns to the left atrial reservoir where it is emptied into the left ventricle, comes out through the aorta and goes back to the lungs again. The net result of the persistence of this fetal shunt is to increase the amount of blood being pumped by the left heart. It increases the work load of the left ventricle and causes an increased blood flow through the lungs. In the course of years, the extra blood going to the lungs can cause permanent damage to the pulmonary arteries.

This birth defect was one of the first to be corrected surgically. Today, it is a simple operation; it is not even necessary for the surgeon to enter the heart—all he does is open the chest, find the persistent little arterial connection between the pulmonary artery and the aorta, tie it off, and sever the communication. When this is done early in life, the heart and great vessels are returned to the normal post-birth state. Such a procedure truly results in curing a birth defect of the heart. Some individuals with very small communications live a normal life-span without correction of the defect.

Another common birth defect is the persistence of a large hole between the right and left atrial reservoirs, or an *atrial septal defect.* Because the pressure is normally higher in the left atrium than in the right atrium, the hole permits oxygenated blood from the left atrium to flow into the right heart. If the defect is very small, the amount of blood shunted through the opening may be inconsequential. The larger the defect, of course, the more mixing between oxygenated and unoxygenated blood will occur. Very large defects can permit unoxygenated blood from the right heart to mix with that coming back from the lungs in the left atrium. In these individuals, the amount of oxygen being carried by the blood leaving the heart is diminished. Very small atrial septal defects may cause minimal or insignificant changes in the function of the heart. Larger ones can seriously compromise its pumping action. Children with fair-sized atrial septal defects often develop slowly and are small and frail, with recurrent episodes of respiratory infections. Today, these defects in the septum can easily be closed, and any such defect of significant size should be corrected.

Some babies are born with a hole in the septum between the right and left ventricular cavities, called a *ventricular septal defect.* Because the pressure is normally higher in the left ventricular cavity than in the right ventricular cavity, such a defect permits oxygenated blood to be shunted from the left heart to the right heart. Under such circumstances, all the blood leaving the left ventricle to the body is normally oxygenated. The abnormal shunting of oxygenated blood to the right ventricle, however, increases the volume in both the right and left ventricular cavities and, if the shunt is large, produces generalized cardiac enlargement. Very small defects of this sort may cause exceptionally loud heart murmurs without significantly increasing the load upon the heart. If the defect is fairly large it can and should be closed.

When open heart surgery became available, more consideration had to be given to the wisdom of closing defects in the ventricular septum. Careful studies of babies with such defects demonstrated that some small openings present at birth normally closed with the growth of the heart. This is one reason why an operation to correct such a defect in very young children might be delayed.

At birth, the pulmonary valve may be deformed and obstructed. Occasionally there will be overgrowth of heart muscle tissue immediately beneath the valve, closing off the outlet from the right ventricle. Such an obstruction, of course, increases the work of the right heart. Severe obstructions can be corrected surgically.

Occasionally an obstruction or constriction of the great aorta will be noted just beyond the heart. Such a defect is called *coarctation of the aorta.* Like any other obstruction to the outflow of blood from the heart, it increases the work of the left ventricular muscle. This defect is more often seen in boys than in girls. After the defect has been recognized it is easily corrected by removing the area of constriction. If the constricted area is only a narrow band, the great aorta may be severed and the ends sewed together. If a longer area of narrowing is observed, the constricted area may be replaced with a graft.

A wide variety of different combinations of these birth defects may be found in any one patient. A baby may have a shunt between the pulmonary artery and the aorta, as well as a hole in the ventricular septum. Sometimes the septal defect in the atria and ventricles are combined. The variety of combinations of such defects, as well as other less common ones, provides a wide spectrum of possible birth defects. Whether or not they should be corrected depends upon their severity and the ease of the operation. Fortunately, the most common defects are the most easily corrected.

Sex and Heart Disease

One of the most important considerations in heart disease is often bypassed—the advisability of sexual activity. Too often the family discusses with the physician all the important aspects of the diet, care of the bowels, how much exercise a patient should receive, and what he should do with his various medications, but the question of sex never arises in the course of these discussions. It must be appreciated that sexual activity produces a vigorous and acute work load upon the circulatory system. Sometimes the first noticeable episodes of chest pain, associated with coronary atherosclerosis, will be noted while participating in the sex act. This is the reason the wise heart specialist will ask his patient if he has any chest discomfort during sexual intercourse. No small number of patients have their first heart attack during sexual intercourse, and still other patients return suddenly to the hospital with a recurrence of chest pain and a new heart attack, caused by premature resumption of vigorous sexual activity soon after their release from the hospital. Clearly, it doesn't make much sense to restrict one's activity to a walk at a leisurely pace down the block, and then to engage in a stress equivalent to a maximum physical effort on a treadmill.

Like all other forms of physical activity, sexual intercourse can be enjoyed without threat to the circulatory system if one has developed the capacity of the heart and circulation so that such events do not represent an acute peak of unusual stress. In normal people sexual intercourse causes major changes in the circulation. The heart rate begins to increase with the excitement phase. There is a lot of truth to the statement that a man's heart rate may increase as he watches a shapely lass walk down the hall. Once the sex act begins, the heart rate and blood pressure in both the male and female increase rapidly. By the time the orgasm is reached, the heart rate may reach levels of between 110 to 180 beats per minute in both men and women. At this juncture it is interesting to note that many investigators studying vigorous young athletes use a heart rate of 180 beats per minute as the cutoff point to stop maximum exertion. During sexual intercourse, along with the increased cardiac output, the systolic blood pressure rises, usually more in men than in women. The rise in blood pressure may be 40 to 100 mmHg. In an individual with a resting systolic blood pressure of 130 mmHg, the systolic blood pressure might be expected to reach levels of 230 mmHg during sexual intercourse. The diastolic pressure is increased by 20 to 50 mmHg. In women, the systolic blood pressure increases 30 to 80 mmHg above its resting level and the diastolic pressure increases 20 to 40 mmHg.

Since systolic blood pressure and heart rate are a good indication of the work being performed by the heart muscle, it is obvious that the increased heart rate and increased systolic blood pressure represent a significant work load for the left ventricular muscle. In an individual with limited blood flow to the heart muscle, these peak work loads can cause angina pectoris. If the activity is sustained too long in certain individuals this may precipitate an acute heart attack. A marked rise in pressure within the heart, coupled with an incompletely healed soft mushy spot in the muscle, can cause the heart to rupture or at best cause poor healing of the damaged area.

Although changes in respiration are not noted in the excitement phases, as soon as sexual activity begins the respiratory rate increases markedly. In both men and women the respiratory rate may rise to forty per minute. The panting, grunting, and respiratory maneuvers that normally occur may influence reflex mechanisms controlling the cardiac rhythm. The reflex actions and the combined work load not infrequently produce a variety of irregularities of the heartbeat, even in individuals without evidence of heart disease.

There is much yet to be learned about the response of the heart and circulatory system to sexual activity. The increase in heart rate and blood pressure, however, does occur regardless of the method of stimulation. It is possible that well-trained sexual partners can control their activity and excitement to diminish peak loads, but it is doubtful that a significant increase in heart rate and blood pressure can be avoided. Sexual intercourse cannot be performed without some excitement and some activity, any more than one can run a mile without running it.

In the vast majority of cases, individuals can resume sexual activity three months after the initial heart attack. But a patient should not expect to go home from the hospital and run on a treadmill, nor should he expect to be able to indulge in vigorous sexual activity. He should gradually get himself back in physical shape to engage in such stressful activity. This means that gradual improvement in physical stamina to the point of being able to jog successfully for a period of ten to fifteen minutes is good insurance against having difficulty during intercourse. In general, sexual activity after a heart attack requiring hospitalization, should probably be postponed for three months after the attack. Much of the first six weeks is often spent in the hospital environment or certainly with markedly limited physical activity. If the first period has gone well, the next six-weeks period should be devoted to gradually increasing physical activity. If there are no difficulties during this three-month period, it is probable that an active sex life can be resumed without undue risk of overloading a weakened heart.

It is important to understand exactly what limitations on sexual activity are imposed by the heart. It is natural that a person who has recovered from a recent heart attack will be concerned about the possibilities of a recurrence. This fear alone may aggravate the condition. In other instances, heart disease provides a convenient excuse for discontinuing an activity that has not been fully satisfactory to one or both marriage partners. The problem here is not heart disease.

An individual with significantly high blood pressure already has a limited capability to increase the work of the heart and circulation. Just as some of these individuals cannot exercise very long on a treadmill, they are also more likely to have difficulties during sexual intercourse. The effect of high blood pressure is to increase the process of atherosclerosis. Accordingly, individuals, particularly men, with high blood pressure are more apt to have heart pain with intercourse than individuals with lower blood pressure.

There are a number of other facets of heart disease that affect sexual activity. Certain drugs given to decrease blood pressure levels have a side effect on the nervous control of the sexual functions. One of these may prevent the male from having a normal ejaculation. Other medications that are used to produce relaxation of constricted arteries to lower blood pressure may prevent the male from developing an adequate erection. Either one of these problems, of course, can be very disturbing to the patient if he doesn't understand them. Anyone who is receiving pills for high blood pressure and has difficulty with sexual activity should discuss the matter frankly with his physician. Often an explanation can be found in the pills that the person is taking and not in the sexuality of the individual.

In some older individuals, the arterial blood supply to the sex organs becomes affected with atherosclerosis and prevents the development of an adequate erection. This complication is frequently accompanied with inadequate arterial blood flow to the legs. Proper surgery, bypassing or correcting the obstruction, often corrects this difficulty.

Some patients have been given a rapid-acting pill by their doctor to relieve fleeting heart pain. These pills are very good for that purpose but they may also have an unfortunate side effect: A man may prepare for sexual intercourse and, knowing from previous experience that he is apt to have chest pain during the activity, take such a pill and place it under his tongue; this may prevent chest pain but very often it will also prevent him from maintaining his erection.

There is no good reason why doctors should be reluctant to discuss these matters with their patients. If a person has any question concerning the relationship of his heart disease to his sex life, or the possible effects of any of the medicines that he may be taking upon his sex life, he should ask these questions of his doctor. A good discussion will go a long way towards relieving a lot of anxiety, and it may provide valuable knowledge that will prevent an unnecessary disaster.

Pregnancy and Heart Disease

Pregnancy increases the work load on the mother's heart. During a normal pregnancy, the mother's blood volume begins to increase after the first three months and may increase as much as thirty per cent by the thirty-second week of pregnancy. The mother's circulation must provide sufficient nutrition and oxygen for herself and the growing baby. Accompanying the increase in the blood volume, the amount of blood pumped by the heart is increased. This, too, begins approximately three months after pregnancy and continues to between the seventh and eighth month of pregnancy. Increased output of blood by the heart is accomplished principally by increasing the resting heart rate. The mother's resting heart rate usually increases ten to twenty beats per minute. The increased volume of blood that must be pumped and the increased heart rate has led to a general estimate that the work of the resting mother's heart may increase as much as fifty per cent by the time of the eighth month of pregnancy.

While increasing the blood volume, it is normal for the mother to retain salt and often fluid. This and pressure factors related to carrying the baby lead to swelling of the feet and ankles, not unlike that noted in heart failure. The increased amount of blood pumped by the heart may set up eddy currents and vibrations responsible for cardiac mumurs. Unless the normal occurrence of these events is appreciated, these findings may be confused with heart failure. To add to the confusion, the mother may experience an increase in palpitations or skipped beats and have shortness of breath during mild exertion or even at rest. The occurrence of such events during pregnancy is not necessarily related to an abnormal function of the heart.

The most common form of heart disease in a young mother is rheumatic heart disease. After all, the complications of coronary atherosclerosis are uncommon in the menstruating female. When rheumatic heart disease is present, this usually means damage to the mitral or aortic valves, or both. This may not significantly influence the course of pregnancy if the valvular damage is minimal. Since damage to either the aortic or mitral valve diminishes the efficiency of the heart muscle's pumping action, it is not surprising that the added stress of pregnancy in a mother with valvular heart disease may cause heart failure. This is the most common complication of pregnancy in a mother with heart disease.

The vast majority of efforts that must be expended by the doctor in supporting a pregnant woman with heart disease is directed toward preventing heart failure. Usually heart failure will not occur until near the fifth month of pregnancy. Thereafter it may get progressively worse until near term. When the blood volume levels off, near the end of pregnancy, and the work of the heart tends to diminish, some relief to the problem of progressively increasing heart failure is offered.

Surprisingly enough, the work load imposed by the pregnancy alone is greater than the work load of labor. For this reason, if a mother has not gone into heart failure prior to delivery, it is not likely that heart failure will occur then. Occasionally heart failure will develop in the days immediately following delivery.

Labor itself is an athletic event. Each contraction of the uterus represents hard work and is accompanied with an increase in blood pressure and heart rate. Between the contractions, the heart rate and blood pressure drop to more normal levels. In general, a mother who has managed to complete her full term of pregnancy and has no other complications will be able to satisfactorily complete delivery.

Knowing that pregnancy is associated with a significant increase in work for the heart muscle, young women with severe heart disease are sometimes discouraged from having babies. Each one of these decisions must be based on a thorough knowledge of the amount of heart disease present. If valvular damage is present and is already taxing the heart muscle to its maximum capability, it is clear that adding the additional load of a fifty per cent increase in cardiac work cannot be achieved. The doctor considers the progressive increase in work load and the ability of the heart to cope with it in an effort to advise his patient concerning the wisdom of future pregnancies. The presence of mild heart disease is seldom a contraindication. The presence of severe heart disease with congestive heart failure usually is sufficient indication to advise against pregnancy. A similar approach is used when considering the influence of less common heart diseases, such as high blood pressure or residual birth defects of the heart. The decision is a complex one and usually requires the considered judgment of both the obstetrician and the heart specialist.

The Truth about Artificial Hearts

Let's face it: The truth is that we do not now have an artificial heart that can be used as a permanent replacement. The concept of an artificial heart is still a dream for the future. One day men will explore Mars and one day permanent artificial hearts will be available, but that day is not now. In most instances, present investigation is directed toward heart assisters, which assist or help with the pumping action of part of the heart on a temporary basis, or the use of a complete artificial heart replacement on a temporary basis. None of these devices helps the person who drops dead from a heart attack.

The development of new complex equipment has enabled physicians to perform operations on the heart that previously were impossible. Only a short time ago, doctors had to limit themselves to tying off the shunt between the aorta and pulmonary artery, when it persisted after birth, or carrying out operations that did not interfere with the continuous pumping action of the heart. The development of the heart-lung machine has enabled the recent major advances in heart surgery. This device can take over the function of the heart and lungs for a short period of time while the heart is opened and operated upon. If the brain is without oxygenated blood for a period of four minutes or longer, significant brain damage or death usually results. This factor has made it impossible for doctors to stop the heart and operate on it directly without resorting to such devices as the heart-lung machine.

Although there are several variations in the way the heart-lung machine can be used, usually the two large venae cavae, returning blood to the right atrium, are tied off and connected in such a way that the venous blood flows directly into the heart-lung machine. As the blood passes through the machine, additional oxygen is added to it in a manner similar to the function of the lungs. Through another connection the oxygenated blood leaving the heart-lung machine is pumped into one or more of the major branches coming directly from the great aorta. In this way, all of the blood coming back from the body is shunted into the machine for oxygenation and then pumped into the arterial system for distribution. Even the coronary arteries to the heart muscle must continue to supply oxygenated blood to the heart tissues or damage to the heart muscle will occur.

When all the appropriate connections are made, the oxygenating function of the lungs and the pumping action of the heart is temporarily replaced by the machine. In this way, it is no longer necessary for respiration to be continued, or for the heart to maintain its pumping action. This provides the doctor with a significant length of time in which to open the heart and to replace diseased valves, such as the aortic valve or mitral valve, or to close a hole in the atrial or ventricular septum. In short, this device has provided the ability to stop the heart long enough to correct any structural abnormalities which may be present. The use of the heart-lung machine has been a dramatic success. There is no question but that it poses some problems, but prior to its use the possibility of stopping the heart for any prolonged period of time, necessary for major heart surgery, was almost nonexistent.

Among the problems which have arisen in using the heart-lung machine is the frequent occurrence of psychosis after the operation. The exact reason for the number of individuals who have temporary psychotic episodes after heart surgery has not been established. Some investigators think it is because of tiny clots and other material that lodge in the brain. Others attribute it directly to the continuous low-pressure output from the heart-lung machine, since the pressure in the arterial system provided by the machine is considerably lower than the systolic pressure usually supplied by the normal heart. Under these circumstances, the more remote tissues may not be receiving enough blood. It is argued that the low pressure level may not provide an adequate blood flow to the brain, causing abnormal function or actual death of many of the brain cells related to personality and intelligence. Fortunately, most patients having this complication after surgery do recover in the course of time. Adequate measurements to detect significant changes in mental function or personality have not yet been accomplished. This is understandable, since prior to the availability of the heart-lung machine, the patients who are now being salvaged were doomed to a downhill course and early death.

Another complication that may follow open heart surgery is impairment or loss of kidney function. This too has raised questions concerning the adequacy of the pressure supplied by the heart-lung machine. In general, the complications of open heart surgery and the heart-lung machine increase sharply the longer the machine has to substitute for the normal function of the heart and lungs. Operations that require stopping the heart only for a short period of time, such as during closure of a hole in the septum between the right and left atrium, usually do not have many complications.

The problems encountered with the use of the heart-lung machine do not detract from the major advances it has permitted. They serve to suggest that further improvements are to be expected in the future and these improvements will significantly advance the quality of heart surgery above the present-day level. The possibility of improved results from heart surgery is one reason that a doctor often recommends postponing heart surgery as long as feasible. He is waiting for the advancements of science to improve his patients' chances of getting a better result with less risk.

The demonstration that it was possible to provide circulation by artificial means kindled the impetus to create an artificial heart. Many scientists recognized that the heart, although it was magnificent, was only a pump. The hope developed and exists today that when the heart was sufficiently damaged its pumping action could be taken over by an artificial device. This, of course, meant that the entire functions of both the right and left heart would have to be assumed by such an artificial mechanism. There are many complex engineering and biological problems to solve before a permanent artificial replacement is developed. One problem is avoiding destruction of the red blood cells, which commonly occurs in the use of artificial devices. Another complication which must be surmounted is the tendency of the blood to develop small clots around implanted artificial devices as has happened in the case of artificial heart valves in many patients. Another difficulty is providing a constant power source for continuous pumping action. The heart is no ordinary pump; the power required to provide continuous pumping generates heat loads and other problems which must be solved before a suitable device is available.

Recognizing these many difficulties, some of the leading heart surgeons addressed their attention to temporary assisters designed to assume only part of the function of the heart. These have been erroneously called *artificial hearts*—they are not. An example of one of these is the type used by a team of physicians at the Texas Medical Center in Houston. The general principles of this device are quite simple. Most commonly it has been used to assist the pumping action of the dominant, or left, ventricle. The increased accumulation of blood in the great left atrial reservoir of the failing heart is passed through a shunt, or tube, from the left atrium to a pump outside the body. Here, through a mechanical device, the blood is entrapped in a pumping chamber and then ejected out of the chamber into another connection to a major artery, usually one in the arm near the chest. The device then taps off the excess blood accumulating behind the failing left ventricle and forces it into the arterial system. In short, it pumps whatever blood the left ventricle is not able to pump. This device is known as the *left ventricular bypass.*

As is customary in the development of circulatory supporting devices, the left ventricular bypass and similar devices have been extensively studied in animal investigation, with considerable success. The same device used in patients with advanced heart disease has not been as satisfactory at this writing. One patient with complete replacement of both the aortic and mitral valves was successfully supported with the left ventricular bypass in the postoperative period and was returned to a relatively normal, productive life. Prior to surgery this patient was severely incapacitated with nothing in the future except a progressive downhill course. This one example is at present the only truly successful result of using the left ventricular bypass in patients with heart disease. The device was used with some success in one other patient, although a residual complication of kidney failure persisted after surgery. All other patients who have been supported on a temporary basis with such a device or similar ones have died in the period immediately following surgery. There is much to be done before a circulatory assister can be of practical benefit in the treatment of heart disease.

All of the problems related to the use of such a device have by no means been solved. Some of the difficulties attributed to the left ventricular bypass device may well be related to the heart-lung machine during surgery. Attaching the left ventricular bypass involves considerable time requiring extended use of the more common heart-lung machine. This may be one of the factors causing serious complications. Another question that remains to be answered is: How much of the pumping function should actually be taken over by the left ventricular bypass device? The optimal approach is yet to be defined. Naturally, the use of the device has been limited to patients with severe advanced heart disease, in whom the outlook was poor. It is possible that these devices may eventually be very helpful in individuals with less severe forms of heart disease. Of course, a more satisfactory approach is to prevent heart disease and prevent the need for such devices.

Another group of artificial devices under development uses the "counterpulsation technique." They also are not intended to replace the heart's function, but to assist the circulation. In the usual device, connections are made directly between the pump and the larger arteries branching directly from the aorta. The purpose of the counterpulsation device is to siphon off blood directly from the aorta when the heart is contracting (systole), and decrease the resistance to ejecting blood from the left heart into the great aorta. In this way the systolic pressure and, consequently, the work of the left ventricular muscle are decreased.

The blood drawn out of the artery into the pump is ejected back into the aorta while the heart muscle is relaxing (diastole). During this phase the aortic valve between the left ventricle and the aorta is closed, so none of the blood runs back into the left ventricular chamber. The injection of blood into the aorta raises the diastolic pressure to cause blood flow throughout the body. Coronary blood flow through the heart muscle is increased. The device thus decreases the work of the left heart while it increases the blood supply and oxygen delivery to the heart muscle. Such a device might be of immense value in an individual with a recent severe heart attack, decreasing the load on the left ventricular muscle and increasing the oxygen supply to the damaged heart muscle.

In April 1969 a giant first step was taken in using the first total artificial replacement of the heart. This historic milestone was achieved by Dr. Denton Cooley, using a device resulting from the work of Dr. Domingo Liotta. The artificial device was used successfully for more than sixty hours in Haskell Karp. It was implanted in the chest and connected to an external power source.

What about the future of artificial circulatory devices? No doubt, better circulatory-assist devices will be developed. Some of the present problems will be solved. The heart-lung machine may be improved, making it easier to install such devices without complications. More knowledge will be gained concerning how best to use these devices in different types of heart patients. Eventually, a complete, permanent artificial heart will be developed. Its use, however, will be limited to medical failures where adequate heart function cannot be expected. The number of individuals falling into this category will progressively decrease. Methods to reconstruct or correct defects in the heart will be improved year by year with the help of better heart-lung machines and circulatory assisters. Better methods of supplying blood to the heart muscle are likely for those individuals who have not developed a successful program to prevent the complications of coronary atherosclerosis.

In most instances, it will be preferable to improve the function of the individual's own heart muscle or improve its blood supply than it will be to make a complete mechanical replacement. *None of these operative procedures will be without risk.* Obviously the preferable solution, whenever possible, will be the prevention of the complications of atherosclerosis or other forms of heart disease, thereby preventing the need for artificial devices, whether they are on a temporary or permanent basis. *The real hope for the future for most people is not the possibility of obtaining an artificial replacement, but of maintaining their present heart in a healthy state.*

New Hearts for Old

The concept of transplanting tissues from one person to another is not new. To the extent that blood may be considered an organ, blood transfusions were the first organ transplants. Early in the history of blood transfusions it was recognized that the blood of some individuals was not compatible with the blood of others. In essence, a form of allergic reaction occurred between two different types of blood. An entire system of *type and cross match* was developed, directly related to classifying an individual's blood type. Blood transfused into a person with a different blood type often resulted in an allergy-like response with clumping end destruction of the red blood cells. Refinements of the methods have developed through the years, until today, most of the problems of blood transfusion have been solved.

In correcting abnormalities of the circulation, the first transplants were replacement of diseased arteries. It was learned that a segment of the great aorta, for example, removed from someone who had died in an automobile accident, could be used to replace a diseased aorta in another patient. There were problems with these grafts, but they did provide a means for the first successful replacements of arteries. Later they were supplanted by synthetic material that could be produced in large amounts and tailored to a variety of lengths or shapes to suit any requirement. These synthetic materials are the primary source for replacement of diseased arteries today.

In more recent times, physicians have been successful in transplanting a kidney or liver from one person to another. Based on these accumulated experiences of transplanting body tissues from one individual to another, a great deal was learned about the body's reactions. In general, if the tissues were not compatible, a form of allergic reaction would develop. The transplanted organ would be considered as an invader. The body's mechanism to develop immunity against such infectious diseases as smallpox or whooping cough is involved in this reaction to a foreign tissue. For these reasons, successful organ transplants have linked surgical skills with increasing knowledge of the body's immune mechanisms and their control. If the immune mechanisms are suppressed, such individuals are susceptible to common infections. On the other hand, if the tissues are not compatible, and the immune mechanisms are not suppressed, the immune allergy-like response will occur, which literally is an attempt to cast off the invading foreign tissue.

The problems attendant to the immune mechanisms have been

resolved sufficiently in recent years that they are often controlled during organ transplants. All of this paved the way for the world's first successful heart transplant. The true complexity of the problem was demonstrated when Dr. Christiaan Barnard performed his first heart transplant at Groote Schuur Hospital, December 3, 1967, on Louis Washkansky. The surgical transplant was apparently accomplished without difficulty. The suppression of the immune mechanism, however, decreased Mr. Washkansky's defenses to the point that he was an easy victim for an overwhelming infection. Nevertheless, the study provided many answers needed to achieve the miracle of human heart transplantation. In a second effort, Dr. Barnard's surgical team carried out a human heart transplant in Dr. Philip Blaiberg on January 2, 1968. This was the world's first successful heart transplant, demonstrating to all the feasibility of human heart transplantation.

The surgery involved in transplanting the heart may be long and tedious but it is not as difficult as some of the other problems previously encountered in reconstruction of the heart. A circular incision is made around the back side of the right atrial reservoir, leaving the two great veins (superior and inferior vena cava) and the back side of the atrium intact. In a similar way, the back side of the left atrial reservoir, with the four main veins draining oxygenated blood back from the lungs, is left in the patient. The back side of the right and left atrial chamber of the donor's heart is then removed. The surgeon sutures the back side of the patient's right and left atria to the donor's heart like two simple circular patches. The recipient's pacemaker, or sparkplug, for the right atrium remains intact, since it normally rests near the entrance of the two great venae cavae into the right atrial reservoir. This means that the control of the pacemaker through the patient's own nervous system is still possible. Other adjustments in rate are made by the automatic mechanisms inherent to the heart itself. Some variations in technique have been used. The famed heart surgeon Dr. Denton Cooley has left both the donor and recipient's pacemaker intact. The pumping action for the entire body is accomplished by the donor's heart. The postoperative dilemma is to prevent rejection of the heart while maintaining the body's immune mechanisms at a sufficient level to avoid an overwhelming infection.

Heart transplants have not yet proved to be very practical. Of the first ninety-five patients receiving transplants, ninety died within five months. This contrasts dramatically with the experience in preventive programs, where the incidence of heart attacks has been decreased by fifty per cent. Adequate preventive programs will go a long way toward obviating the need for extensive use of either artificial devices or organ transplants.

What to Do When the Circulation Fails

With the increased frequency of heart attacks, sooner or later you will probably be confronted with an individual whose circulation has stopped. This usually occurs when no doctor or other medical assistance is available. If you know what to do, you may well be able to save someone's life. The simple truth is, today the necessity to provide artificial circulation is greater than the necessity to provide artificial respiration. There are far more victims of heart attacks than of drowning. Of course, one must be certain that adequate respiration is occurring when artificial circulation is given.

Heart attacks have no particular respect for the time of their occurrence. They may occur at the end of a sumptuous meal, either at home or in a restaurant, or they may occur at public gatherings. In almost every instance, someone is with the individual or immediately available when the heart attack occurs. Because of the sensitivity of the brain to a lack of oxygen, artificial circulation must be effected within four minutes after the circulation has stopped, otherwise the victim may have severe and permanent brain damage.

The circulation may stop, either because the heart has stopped beating (cardiac arrest) or because the rhythm of death (ventricular fibrillation) occurs. In either case, the effective pumping action of the heart muscle stops. It is not necessary to determine which mechanism has caused the circulation to stop before providing artificial circulation.

If you are in a situation where someone suddenly collapses, first find out if the person is still breathing. If the respiration has stopped, proceed as follows:

1. Lay the victim on his back on a hard surface—the floor is fine; do not use a bed. Tilt the head back so that the neck is straight. Be sure the mouth is clear of food or obstruction.
2. Pinch the nose shut with your fingers and keep it shut. Put

your mouth over the victim's and exhale into it. The victim's chest should expand as it does in normal breathing unless there is an obstruction in the airway (trachea or windpipe). In the case of a small child your mouth can cover both the mouth and nose.

3. Remove your mouth, and the victim's lungs will automatically exhale the air you breathed into his lungs.
4. Repeat three or four breaths—sometimes respiration will begin spontaneously.

In the event that a mechanical airway, such as a plastic tube, is available it should be inserted down behind the tongue of the victim and into the windpipe (this is the first opening directly be-

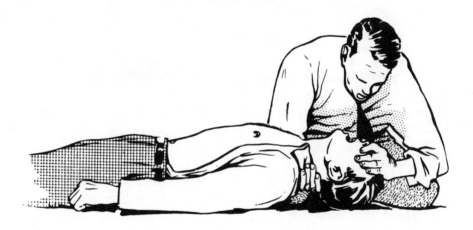

hind the tongue). The other end of the tube protrudes from the victim's mouth enabling you to provide artificial respiration with your mouth, proceeding as previously described.

A plastic tube is relatively inexpensive, and considering the frequent need for such a device, one should be present in all public places beside the fire extinguisher. Public awareness of this need has not yet been stimulated; consequently, when someone has an acute collapse in a public place, such a simple inexpensive device—which can be lifesaving—is not available. Obviously it is much

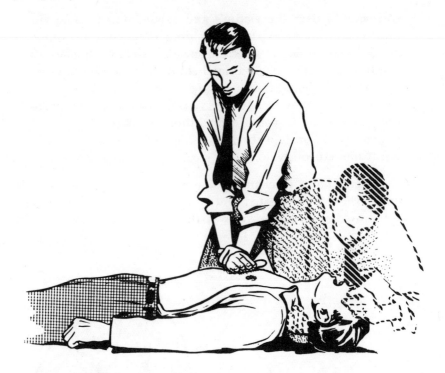

easier to get someone to use such a mechanical airway than to per-form mouth-to-mouth respiration if the victim is a stranger.

Now direct your attention to the circulation as follows:

1. Find out whether the victim has a pulse or not. You can try several locations and if you feel a pulse at any of these places you need not give artificial circulation, but should continue artificial respiration (fifteen breaths per minute) as long as it is needed. Feel the wrist above the thumb. Feel the temple just in front of the ear. Feel the neck just below the jaw. Feel the chest just below the left breast. If no pulse is felt you should assume circulation has stopped.

2. Try to start the heart beating by striking a sharp blow with your fist just to the left of the breastbone (sternum) and below the nipple. Check for a pulse again. If the heart has not started, strike the chest again.

3. If the above procedure fails to start the heart you must provide artificial circulation.

    a. Get down on your knees, facing the victim.

b. Place the heel of one hand directly on the lower part of the sternum just above the pit of the stomach (your hand must be on the breastbone—not over the stomach).

c. Place the other hand on top of the hand on the victim's lower sternum.

d. Keeping the elbows straight, rise up and then apply a downward pressure, directly upon the sternum. The effective pressure in an adult is about seventy pounds, or enough to push the sternum down toward the backbone about two inches. The downward compression of the sternum compresses the heart, squeezing blood out of the heart into the arterial circulation.

e. Immediately after you have exerted downward pressure on the sternum, release the pressure, allowing the sternum to snap back to its original position. During this period, the heart refills with blood.

f. This procedure should be repeated continuously, replacing the normal beating of the heart. The rate should approximate the normal heartbeat, about sixty times a minute. A good way to do the procedure is to count while exerting the pressure. As you rise forward and press down on the sternum, count one-thousand-one, maintaining the downward pressure momentarily for the count of one, then releasing it. Repeat the procedure counting one-thousand-two, maintaining the downward pressure for the count of two, one-thousand-three, one-thousand-four, one-thousand-five, and so on until you reach one-thousand-ten; then start the count again at one-thousand-one, one-thousand-two, etc. This provides a fairly rhythmic way of being certain that you are causing one downward stroke each second. If you supply sufficient downward pressure, this method frequently will maintain adequate pumping action for a marginal but satisfactory circulation.

4. About every twenty seconds you should stop, close off the nostrils, and again exhale three times into the lungs of the victim. Obviously if you have a partner present, he can provide artificial respiration on a continuous basis of fifteen breaths per minute.

It is apparent that if the lungs are not adequately ventilated, the blood circulated to the lungs by chest compression will not be oxygenated and there will be no point in providing artificial circulation.

Fortunately, in a certain number of individuals, soon after the procedure is begun, normal heart action may return. Periodically check to see if the pulse can be felt in any of the locations previously mentioned. If the heartbeat returns and respiration is normal, the victim should be left lying comfortably until medical assistance can.be obtained.

In the case of babies and small children, the method of providing external massage must be modified. In small children, the fingers of each hand can be wrapped around the back with the thumbs placed directly on the middle of the sternum, somewhat higher than the location recommended for adults. External pressure is then produced with the thumbs, being careful not to overcompress the sternum but still attempting to provide a movement of one or two inches. Other modifications may be necessary depending upon the size of the victim, but the principle is still the same— downward compression of the sternum at regular intervals while maintaining adequate respiration.

It is true that you can create damage by the improper use of artificial circulation. The most common damage is fracturing the ribs connected to the sternum, tearing the liver, or causing a tear in the lung. If you are careful not to use excessive amounts of pressure, these problems are not likely to occur. While such complications are unfortunate, it is much better to have received artificial circulation and sustained a few broken ribs or even a torn lung or liver, than to have died intact.

If you are present when the circulation stops, remember you can do something while you are waiting for the doctor, and you have less than four minutes to do it. If every American were aware of this simple procedure and had carefully rehearsed and memorized the mechanics, a substantial number of individuals who arrive at the emergency room dead on arrival would have an opportunity to receive medical assistance. If your friends and family knew how to accomplish this procedure, the life they save could be yours.

The American Heart Association's
Fat-Controlled, Low-Cholesterol Meal Plan

THIS PLAN is mainly for adults from their twenties on who have a family history of heart disease, or who may have increased their risks through a regular diet high in saturated fat and cholesterol. Children and adolescents, especially from susceptible families, can also benefit from this meal plan by forming tastes for food early in life that may protect them from heart disease when they reach adulthood.

The *types* of food recommended here are suitable for most people from childhood through maturity. The *amounts* of food specified in the food lists, however, are recommended mainly for the average adult. Nutritional needs differ during growth periods of infants, children, and adolescents, and during pregnancy and breast feeding; at these times, the amounts of food to be eaten should be regulated by a physician.

Every day, select foods from each of the basic food groups in lists 1–5, and follow the recommendations for number and size of servings.

1 *Meat, Poultry, Fish, Dried Beans and Peas, Nuts, Eggs*

1 serving: 3–4 ounces of cooked meat or fish (not including bone or fat) or 3–4 ounces of a vegetable listed here. Use 2 or more servings (a total of 6–8 ounces) daily.

Recommended

Chicken · **turkey** · **veal** · **fish** · in most of your meat meals for the week.

Beef · **lamb** · **pork** · **ham** · in no more than 5 meals per week. Choose lean ground meat and lean cuts of meat · trim all visible fat before cooking · bake, broil, roast, or stew so that you can discard the fat which cooks out of the meat.

Nuts and dried beans and peas: Kidney beans · lima beans · baked beans · lentils · chick peas *(garbanzos)* · split peas · are high in vegetable protein and may be used in place of meat occasionally.

Egg whites as desired.

Avoid or Use Sparingly

Duck · goose.

Shellfish: clams · crab · lobster · oysters · scallops · shrimp · are low in fat but high in cholesterol. Use a 4-ounce serving in a meat meal no more than once a week.

Heavily marbled and fatty meats · spare ribs · mutton · frankfurters · sausages · fatty hamburgers · bacon · luncheon meats.

Organ meats: liver · kidney · heart · sweetbreads · are very high in cholesterol. Since liver is very rich in vitamins and iron, it should not be eliminated from the diet completely. Use a 4-ounce serving in a meat meal no more than once a week.

Egg yolks: limit to 3 per week, including eggs used in cooking.

Cakes, batters, sauces, and other foods containing egg yolks.

2 *Vegetables and Fruit*

(FRESH, FROZEN, OR CANNED)

1 serving: ½ cup. Use at least 4 servings daily.

Recommended

One serving should be a source of vitamin C:
Broccoli • cabbage (raw) • tomatoes.

Berries • cantaloupe • grapefruit (or juice) • mango • melon • orange (or juice) • papaya • strawberries • tangerines.

One serving should be a source of vitamin A—dark green leafy or yellow vegetables, or yellow fruits:
Broccoli • carrots • chard • chicory • escarole • greens (beet, collard, dandelion, mustard, turnip) • kale • peas • rutabagas • spinach • string beans • sweet potatoes and yams • watercress • winter squash • yellow corn.

Apricots • cantaloupe • mango • papaya.

Other vegetables and fruits are also very nutritious; they should be eaten in salads, main dishes, snacks, and desserts, *in addition* to the recommended daily allowances of high vitamin A and C vegetables and fruits. If you must limit your calories, use a serving of potatoes, yellow corn, or fresh or frozen cooked lima beans in place of a bread serving.

Avoid or Use Sparingly

Olives and avocados are very high in fat calories and should be used in moderation.

3 Bread and Cereals

(WHOLE GRAIN, ENRICHED, OR RESTORED)

1 serving of bread: 1 slice. 1 serving of cereal: ½ cup, cooked; 1 cup, cold, with skimmed milk. Use at least 4 servings daily.

Recommended

Breads made with a minimum of saturated fat:
White enriched (including raisin bread) • whole wheat • English muffins • French bread • Italian bread • oatmeal bread • pumpernickel • rye bread.

Biscuits, muffins, and griddle cakes made at home, using an allowed liquid oil as shortening.

Cereal (hot and cold) • rice • melba toast • matzo • pretzels.

Pasta: macaroni • noodles (except egg noodles) • spaghetti.

Avoid or Use Sparingly

Butter rolls • commercial biscuits, muffins, doughnuts, sweet rolls, cakes, crackers • egg bread, cheese bread • commercial mixes containing dried eggs and whole milk.

4 *Milk Products*

1 serving: 8 ounces (1 cup). **Daily servings of skimmed milk (fortified with vitamins A and D) for children under 9: 2–3 cups; for children 9–12: 3 or more cups; for teen-agers: 4 or more cups; for adult: 2 or more cups.**

Recommended

Milk products that are low in dairy fats:

Fortified skimmed (non-fat) milk and fortified skimmed milk powder • low-fat milk. The label on the container should show that the milk is fortified with vitamins A and D. The word "fortified" alone is not enough.

Buttermilk made from skimmed milk • yogurt made from skimmed milk • canned evaporated skimmed milk • cocoa made with low-fat milk.

Cheeses made from skimmed or partially skimmed milk, such as cottage cheese, creamed or uncreamed (uncreamed, preferably) • farmer's, baker's or hoop cheese • mozarella and sapsago cheeses made with partially skimmed milk.

Avoid or Use Sparingly

Whole milk and whole milk products:

Chocolate milk • canned whole milk • ice cream • all creams including sour, half and half, whipped • whole milk yogurt.

Nondairy cream substitutes (usually contain coconut oil).

Cheeses made from cream or whole milk.

Butter.

5 *Fats and Oils*

(POLY-UNSATURATED)

An individual allowance should include about 2–4 tablespoons daily (depending on how many calories you can afford) in the form of margarine, salad dressing, and shortening.

Recommended

Margarines, liquid oil shortenings, salad dressings, and mayonnaise containing any of these poly-unsaturated vegetable oils: Corn oil • cottonseed oil • safflower oil • sesame seed oil • soybean oil • sunflower-seed oil.

Margarines and other products high in poly-unsaturates can usually be identified by their label which lists a recommended *liquid* vegetable oil as the *first* ingredient, and one or more partially hydrogenated vegetable oils as additional ingredients.

Diet margarines are low in calories because they are low in fat. Therefore it takes twice as much diet margarine to supply the poly-unsaturates contained in a recommended margarine.

Avoid or Use Sparingly

Solid fats and shortenings: Butter • lard • salt pork fat • meat fat • completely hydrogenated margarines and vegetable shortenings.

Peanut oil and olive oil may be used occasionally for flavor, but they are low in poly-unsaturates and do not take the place of the recommended oils.

6 *Desserts, Beverages, Snacks, Condiments*

The foods on this list are acceptable because they are low in saturated fat and cholesterol. If you have eaten your daily allowance from the first five lists, however, these foods will be in excess of your nutritional needs, and many of them also may exceed your calorie limits for maintaining a desirable weight. If you must limit your calories, limit your portions of the foods on this list as well.

Moderation should be observed especially in the use of alcoholic drinks, ice milk, sherbet, sweets, and bottled drinks.

Acceptable

Low in calories or no calories:
Fresh fruit and fruit canned without sugar • tea, coffee (no cream), cocoa powder • water ices • gelatin • fruit whip • puddings made with non-fat milk • sweets and bottled drinks made with artificial sweeteners • vinegar, mustard, ketchup, herbs, spices.

High in calories:
Frozen or canned fruit with sugar added • jelly, jam, marmalade, honey • pure sugar candy such as gum drops, hard candy, mint patties (not chocolate) • imitation ice cream made with safflower oil • cakes, pies, cookies, and puddings made with poly-unsaturated fat in place of solid shortening • angel food cake • nuts, especially walnuts • nonhydrogenated peanut butter • bottled drinks • fruit drinks • ice milk • sherbet • wine, beer, whisky.

Avoid or Use Sparingly

Coconut and coconut oil • commercial cakes, pies, cookies, and mixes • frozen cream pies • commercially fried foods such as potato chips and other deep fried snacks • whole milk puddings • chocolate pudding (high in cocoa butter and therefore high in saturated fat) • ice cream.

Index